SEXUAL ANOREXIA

"In *Sexual Anorexia: Overcoming Sexual Self-Hatred,* Patrick Carnes explores more of the continuum of human sexual dysfunction. With all the moral injunctions about sex that most of us received during childhood, it is difficult to see a lack of, or even revulsion of, sexual desire as a serious problem. In comparing these areas of difficulty with the anorexic and bulimic eating disorders, Carnes masterfully presents an easily understood structure of the disease process and a recovery regime that offers real hope for comfort in relationships."

—Pia Mellody, R.N., addictions and codependence consultant, author of *Facing Codependence, Breaking Free,* and *Facing Love Addiction*

"A valuable resource for men and women who have been afraid and confused about sex. Patrick Carnes has made another remarkable contribution that fosters sexual recovery and sexual healing. Using his trademark blend of wisdom, practical strategies, and personal stories, Carnes takes readers through a step-by-step program to discover the meaning and joys of healthy sexual intimacy."

—Wendy Maltz, M.S.W., sex therapist, author of *The Sexual Healing Journey* and co-author of *In the Garden of Desire*

SEXUAL ANOREXIA

Overcoming

Sexual

Self-Hatred

Patrick Carnes, Ph.D.
with Joseph M. Moriarity

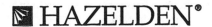 HAZELDEN®

INFORMATION & EDUCATIONAL SERVICES

Hazelden
Center City, Minnesota 55012-0176

1-800-328-0094 (Toll Free U.S., Canada, and the Virgin Islands)
1-651-257-1331 (24-hour Fax)
http://www.hazelden.org (World Wide Web site on Internet)

©1997 by Patrick Carnes. Printed in the United States of America. No portion of this publication may be reproduced in any manner without the written permission of the publisher

Library of Congress Cataloging-in-Publication Data
Carnes, Patrick
 Sexual anorexia: overcoming sexual self-hatred/Patrick Carnes.
 p. cm.
 Includes bibliographical references and index.
 ISBN 1-56838-144-1
 1. Sexual aversion disorders. I. Title.
RC560.S45C37 1997   97-12610
616.85'83—dc21   CIP

05 04 03 02 01 6 7 8 9 10

Book design by Nora Koch/Gravel Pit Publications
Cover design by David Spohn
Typesetting by Nora Koch/Gravel Pit Publications

Editor's note
Hazelden offers a variety of information on chemical dependency and related areas. Our publications do not necessarily represent Hazelden's programs, nor do they officially speak for any Twelve Step organization.

All the stories in this book are based on actual experiences. The names and details have been changed to protect the privacy of the people involved. In some cases, composites have been created.

The Twelve Steps are reprinted with permission of Alcoholics Anonymous World Services, Inc. Permission to reprint and adapt the Twelve Steps does not mean that AA has reviewed or approved the contents of this publication, nor that AA agrees with the views expressed herein. AA is a program of recovery from alcoholism *only*—use of the Twelve Steps in connection with programs and activities which are patterned after AA, but which address other problems, or in any other non-AA context, does not imply otherwise.

This book is dedicated to the couples who participate in Recovering Couples Anonymous.

CONTENTS

ILLUSTRATIONS

Figures

Preface

In many ways, this book began in 1983 when I completed *Out of the Shadows: Understanding Sexual Addiction*. That book described the nature of sexual addiction and the path of recovery from the illness. Yet I knew even then that *Out of the Shadows* told only part of the story. From that point on, I tried to define sexual addiction as part of a continuum. On one end were people who had lost the ability to regulate their own sexual behavior. On the other extreme were those who could not force themselves to be sexual without dire internal consequences. The two conditions were related. Both obsessional states drew their power from a deep sexual self-hatred.

In 1989, I completed *Contrary to Love*, which described sexual addiction for professionals. The book began with the continuum of compulsive sex and compulsive nonsex. It also described in detail how sex addicts go through periods of "deescalation" in which "sex becomes the enemy." The whole process of therapy and recovery is directed toward sexual health, which at that point I only partly defined.

Since then, we have witnessed a decade of extraordinary progress. Twelve Step groups for sexual addiction, such as Sex and Love Addicts Anonymous, Sexaholics Anonymous, Sex Addicts Anonymous, and Sexual Compulsives Anonymous, have flourished across the country and throughout the world. The National Council on Sexual Addiction and Compulsivity is in its fourth year of publishing a medical journal dedicated to the problem. Inpatient and outpatient programs for sexual addiction have sprung up across the nation. In 1997, three basic medical texts included chapters on sexual addiction.

In the midst of rapidly expanding awareness about sexual addiction, a growing consciousness about what I call sexual anorexia has also emerged—albeit more slowly. Twelve Step groups held conferences, published literature, and offered groups to sexual anorexics. The concern was more tentative for sexual anorexia, however, in part because the losses are more hidden. But professionals began to note the connections between sexual acting out and "acting in." Those who researched abuse, especially sexual abuse, wrote about "traumatic abstinence." Sexologists separated sexual aversion as a more extreme problem than sexual dysfunction. And like the addiction specialists, they now acknowledged a continuum of extremes. Yet no one book defined the problem for those seeking recovery using a Twelve Step format. There was no *Out of the Shadows* for the sexual anorexic.

Another problem also started to reveal itself. As I traveled and spoke about recovery, I heard many people ask, "What is healthy sexuality?" In 1991, I wrote more about that in *Don't Call It Love*, wherein I described eight dimensions of healthy sexuality. These specific dimensions grew out of the research for that book, which involved interviewing over one thousand recovering sex addicts and their partners. I used the model of the eight dimensions in my speeches and workshops. In one such workshop, it dawned on me that the workshop participants already possessed the tools for understanding what it was they sought. Those tools were the very Twelve Step principles with which they were already familiar in other contexts. Recovering people simply needed to know that they could apply their Twelve Step skills to their sexuality. When I spoke around the country, I could see how helpful making that bridge was. People started to use the materials, and soon *Sexual Anorexia: Overcoming Sexual Self-Hatred* started to take form. Once I realized how the principles of the Twelve Steps paralleled the dimensions of healthy sexuality, I expanded the latter from eight to twelve. A matrix matching the (now) twelve dimensions with twelve supportive strategies for achieving them and the applicable principles of the Twelve Steps can be found in appendix A. This matrix provides a quick overview of what this book hopes to accomplish and how to get there.

Sexual Anorexia fills in the parts for which *Out of the Shadows* only sketched the outlines. In addition to creating a method for exploring healthy sexuality, this book completes the picture of what sexual anorexia looks like. It also draws connections with sexual addiction and other excessive or deprivation behaviors. In that sense, it might be a bit unsettling for those who like to keep their addiction and compulsive disorders in neat, separate categories. Inpatient providers as well as outpatient therapists now understand that these extremes interact with one another and that, unless the whole web of compulsions and addictions is addressed, the web will continually reanchor itself in some new self-destructive constellation.

Sexual anorexia and sexual addiction are but two of the anchor sites available to the addictive-compulsive process. Thus, when I refer in the book to "treatment centers," I am referring to those therapeutic institutions that in some manner treat addictions or compulsions. I am speaking most specifically, however, of those organizations that recognize, understand, and in some manner provide services to address the complex interrelation of addictive disorders. One such institution is the Meadows, in Wickenburg, Arizona, where I do my clinical work as a therapist with sex addicts and anorexics in and across the spectrum of addiction, depression, trauma, and various phobias. Thus, although this book focuses primarily on the sexual anorexic and his or her partner, it can be used as well by anyone in any type of recovery program who decides to confront and begin healing sexual issues.

Acknowledgments

I am grateful to the clinical staff of the Meadows, the treatment center where I do my clinical work. It is truly one of the institutions that understands the "web" and the constellations of addictive and emotional disorders. The staff were quick to incorporate anorexia First Steps into their work with clients suffering from sexual and other addictions, trauma, and depression. I particularly want to thank Maureen Canning and the primary counselors, the family counseling staff, and nursing staff. Jeanne Hawks, my office manager, has been a great gift to me in helping with the manuscript as well as keeping the "affairs of state" going when I have been writing. Pat Mellody, the executive director of the Meadows, made much of the book possible by providing resources, by believing in and supporting what I do, and by committing himself to the field of addiction recovery.

I want to thank the recovering people who generously shared their stories for this book. Many of them were members of Recovering Couples Anonymous (RCA). As a fellowship focused on couples, RCA is founded on a clear understanding of the web addiction as it affects families. I appreciate how RCA groups have used my work in their meetings. I have substantially altered details of the stories that appear in this book in order to preserve the anonymity of RCA members.

I have often been impatient with myself over my writing. *Out of the Shadows* took ten years to finish and publish. This book also represents a decade of efforts. When Hazelden explained to me the time line for finishing the book, I was in the midst of moving to the Meadows from the hospital where I'd worked previously. The task was then to write while moving. Fortunately, I had the assistance of Joseph Moriarity who took my notes and ideas and helped me fashion many of the chapters in this book. In addition to actually crafting the prose of the last twelve chapters, he provided research assistance and conducted several interviews. We had many late nights together, which made

Acknowledgments

me appreciate his competence, judgment, and great kindness. Without his strong work ethic and his support, finishing this book would have been an impossible task. Also I cannot say enough about Steve Lehman and Dan Odegard of Hazelden who gave me editorial support far beyond what is normal. I am deeply grateful for their faith in me as well.

Many colleagues have supported me over the years in this work in looking at sexual help. They include Martha Turner, Sherry Sedgewick, Cheryl Campbell, Sharon Nathan, Richard Irons, Carol Thompson, Judith Matheney, Ken Adams, Gerald Blanchard, Colleen Land, and Rip Corlee. I want also to acknowledge Ginger Manley, a sexologist who pioneered the promotion of sexual health for sex addicts. Another special colleague is trauma specialist Wendy Maltz, whose work in sexual recovery for abuse victims is landmark. Their encouragement in our writing has been key to bringing this book to light.

Finally, I wish to thank my wife, Suzanne. The quiet intimacy we share has been a refuge to me during the writing of this book. The degree that this book conveys peace and care reflects how she is and how we are together.

For information on therapists in your local area, please call 1-800-632-3697. For information on workshops, conferences, and retreats with Dr. Carnes, please call 1-800-621-4062, or write the Meadows, 1655 N. Tegner St., Wickenburg, AZ 85390. For information on audio- and videotapes as well as other publications by Dr. Carnes, call 1-800-955-9853, or write New Freedom Publications, P.O. Box 3345, Wickenburg, AZ 85358.

INTRODUCTION

They suffer silently, consumed by a dread of sexual pleasure and filled with fear and sexual self-doubt. They feel profoundly at odds with a culture that tirelessly promotes sex but is strangely unconscious about sexuality. It is not inhibited sexual desire they are experiencing, although often they possess a naiveté, an innocence, or even a prejudice against sex. It is not sexual dysfunction, although their suffering often wears the mask of physical problems that affect sex. It is not about being cold and unresponsive although that certainly is a way in which they protect themselves against the hurt. It is not about religious belief, although religious sexual oppression may have been a place to hide. It is not about guilt and shame, although those feelings are powerfully experienced. Nor is it about sexual betrayal or risk or rejection, although those are common themes. It is simply the emptiness of profound deprivation, a silent suffering called sexual anorexia.

Sexual anorexia is an obsessive state in which the physical, mental, and emotional task of avoiding sex dominates one's life. Like self-starvation with food or compulsive debting or hoarding with money, deprivation with sex can make one feel powerful and defended against all hurts. As with any other altered state of consciousness, such as those brought on by chemical use, compulsive gambling or eating, or any other addiction process, the preoccupation with the avoidance of sex can seem to obliterate one's life problems. The obsession can then become a way to cope with all stress and all life difficulties. Yet, as with other addictions and compulsions, the costs are great. In this case, sex becomes a furtive enemy to be continually kept at bay, even at the price of annihilating a part of oneself.

The word anorexia comes from the Greek word *orexis*, meaning appetite. An-orexis, then, means the denial of appetite. When referring to food appetite, anorexia means the obsessive state of food avoidance that translates into self-starvation. Weight concerns and fear of fat transform into a hatred of food and a hatred of the body because the body demands the nurturance of food. Food anorexics perceive bodily cravings for sustenance as a failure of self-discipline. The refusal to eat also becomes a way for food anorexics to reassert power against others, particularly those who may be perceived as trying to control the anorexic, trying in some manner to prevent the anorexic from being his or her "true" self. Ironically, many food anorexics are driven by a powerful need to meet unreal cultural standards about the attractiveness of being thin. A terror of sexual rejection rules their thoughts and behaviors and is a primary force behind this striving for thinness. The irony here is that sexual anorexics share precisely the same terror.

Specialists in sexual medicine have long noted the close parallels between food disorders and sexual disorders. Many professionals have observed how food anorexia and sexual anorexia share common characteristics.[1] In both cases, the sufferers starve themselves in the midst of plenty. Both types of anorexia feature the essential loss of self, the same distortions of thought, and the agonizing struggle for control over the self and others. Both share the same extreme self-hatred and sense of profound alienation. But while the food anorexic is obsessed with the self-denial of physical nourishment, the sexual anorexic focuses his or her anxiety on sex. As a result, the sexual anorexic will typically experience the following:

- a dread of sexual pleasure
- a morbid and persistent fear of sexual contact
- obsession and hypervigilance around sexual matters
- avoidance of anything connected with sex
- preoccupation with others being sexual
- distortions of body appearance
- extreme loathing of body functions
- obsessional self-doubt about sexual adequacy

- rigid, judgmental attitudes about sexual behavior
- excessive fear and preoccupation with sexually transmitted diseases
- obsessive concern or worry about the sexual intentions of others
- shame and self-loathing over sexual experiences
- depression about sexual adequacy and functioning
- intimacy avoidance because of sexual fear
- self-destructive behavior to limit, stop, or avoid sex

Sexual anorexics can be men as well as women. Their personal histories often include sexual exploitation or some form of severely traumatic sexual rejection—or both. Experiences of childhood sexual abuse are common with sexual anorexics, often accompanied by other forms of childhood abuse and neglect. As a result of these traumas, they may tend to carry dark secrets and maintain seemingly insane loyalties that have never been disclosed. In fact, sexual anorexics are for the most part not conscious of the hidden dynamics driving them. Although obsessed with sexual avoidance, they are nonetheless also prone to sexual bingeing—occasional periods of extreme sexual promiscuity, or "acting out"—in much the way that bulimics will binge with compulsive overeating and then purge by self-induced vomiting. Sexual anorexics may also compensate with other extreme behaviors such as chemical or behavioral addictions, co-dependency, or deprivation behaviors like debting, hoarding, saving, cleaning, or various phobic responses. The families of sexual anorexics may also present extreme patterns of behavior and thought. Finally, the sexual anorexic is likely to have been deeply influenced by a cultural, social, or religious group that views sex negatively and supports sexual oppression and repression.

Sexual anorexia, therefore, can wear many masks. Consider the sexual trauma victim who takes care of her pain by compulsively overeating. People focus on her obesity, not noticing the hidden anorexic agenda of avoiding being desirable to anyone. Or think of the alcoholic who has never been sexual except when drinking. The prospect of being sexual while sober is so intimidating that a broader "abstinence" is embraced. For most sexual anorexics, however, a complex array of extremes exists. When a person's appetites are excessive we use words like addiction or compulsion. But excesses are often accompanied by extreme deprivations for which we use terms like anorexia or obsession. In fact, these seemingly mutually exclusive states can exist simultaneously within a person and within a family. Consider the case of a sexually addicted alcoholic heterosexual male. The further his drinking and sexual behavior get out of control, the harder and more compulsively his wife works (the more she behaves hyper-responsibly), and the more she shuts down sexually (anorexia). These disorders are not occurring in isolation. But the end result is that the problem of sexual anorexia is not likely to get addressed because it lacks the clarity and drama of the drinking, the sexual acting out, and the workaholism.

People minimize the problem of sexual anorexia. After all, whoever died of a lack of sex? Yet, as we shall see in this book, the physical and psychological consequences of sexual anorexia are severe, and the problem is central to understanding the entire mosaic of extreme behaviors.

This book focuses on the suffering of the sexual anorexic. Sexual anorexia is as destructive as the illnesses that often accompany it, and behind which it often hides, such as alcoholism, drug addiction, sexual addiction, and compulsive eating. It resides in emotion so raw that most sufferers would wish to keep it buried forever were it not so painful to live this way. Sexual anorexia feeds on betrayal, violence, and rejection. It gathers strength from a culture that makes sexual satisfaction both an unreachable goal and a nonnegotiable demand. Our media focus almost exclusively on sensational sexual problems such as rape, child abuse, sexual harassment, or extramarital affairs. When people have problems being sexual, we are likely to interpret the difficulty as a need for a new technique or a matter of misinformation. For those who suffer from sexual anorexia, technique and information are not remotely enough. Help comes only through an intentional, planned effort to break the bonds of obsession that keep anorexics stuck.

This book is intended as a guide to support that effort. The early chapters help the reader understand sexual anorexia: how it starts, and how it gathers such strength. The last twelve chapters present a clinically tested and proven plan for achieving a healthy sexuality. This program has worked for many, many people. It is safe. It is practical. It works if the sufferer follows the guidelines and has the appropriate outside support. It will not be easy because the obsession was created in the first place by intimate violations and shattered trust. Yet step by step, healing can be effected so that the sufferer can learn to trust the self as well as others.

The plan is designed to involve a network of external support made up of partners, therapists, close friends, clergy, and so on. The book will explain the importance of having these "fair witnesses" along on the journey to health and freedom. Breaking the isolation is essential to dismantling the dysfunctional beliefs and loyalties that keep people in pain.

The material in this book can be used in many settings. Some people have used these materials in the Twelve Step groups dedicated to sexual problems, many of which now feature subgroups dedicated to sexual anorexia. Couples groups dedicated to recovery such as Recovering Couples Anonymous have also used these materials as a guide. Therapists have used them in individual and group therapeutic sessions.

Many observers, including myself, have noticed that sexual anorexics are generally competent and willing people. As they face their illness, they begin to reclaim their creativity and start becoming the persons they were meant to be. There is something fundamental about coming to terms with the sexual self, something healing and liberating. In the "Big Book" of Alcoholics Anonymous one of the promises of recovery is "we shall know a new freedom!" This book is dedicated to making that so.

PART

I

SEX AS FUNDAMENTAL

Appetite (for food) and sexual drive are related. . . . One is not merely a displacement, symbolization, or substitution for the other. Rather, appetite and sexual drive are related but distinct parts of a constellation of bodily urges that the holy anorexic seeks to tame and ultimately to obliterate.

—Rudolph M. Bell

Holy Anorexia

CAROL HATED DISHONESTY. Nothing had hurt her more than other people's lies. Yet she had a terrible secret that she knew would hurt her husband. And the moment had arrived when she knew she had to tell him. The two of them were sitting with their therapist, Miriam. This lovely, wise therapist had seen many couples over her thirty years as a clinician. She surmised that Carol and Chet knew very little about each other's history. They thought they knew, but they did not. As a result, they were struggling as a couple and as individuals. Miriam had asked Chet and Carol to share in detail their individual family histories and their relationship history. Chet had just finished his story of childhood sexual abuse, which was very difficult to hear. In part, it was the sheer pain of his experience that was hard to listen to. Yet, also, there were some startling revelations, the implications of which were stunning. Carol was the first to see fully what her therapist already intuitively knew. They had been living an extraordinary lie. And now it was her turn. If she were truthful, the fullness of the deceit would become apparent.

When Carol and Chet started their relationship, it was instantly sexual. In fact, they would often talk about how good the sex was—despite all the other problems they had as a couple. They now had two small sons and even their births had not stopped their desire—even if they now had somewhat less opportunity. Chet said a number of times that he was lucky to have a woman so willing. Carol never refused him. Yet therein was part of the lie: Carol hated her sexuality and detested being sexual. She had long believed that to have a husband and family, she had to be sexual. Every orgasm and every sexual initiative she had taken over nine years of courtship and marriage had been faked. The only genuine orgasms she had experienced were in a very complicated ritual in the bathtub in which she used the stream of water from the faucet to stimulate herself. And she could only achieve that when alone. Everything else was a sham.

Carol had hated her sexuality ever since she was a child. This feeling was usually connected to being with her dad. He would comment on her body, about how cute it was, and say she was growing up nicely. She liked her father's attention and liked to cuddle with him. Yet, when he would cheer her skimpy bathing suits (which were probably inappropriately brief for her age) or express disappointment when she put street clothes back on, she felt very uneasy. When Carol and her three sisters were little, her father had taken lots of pictures of them in the bathtub with no clothes on. Seeing these photos as an adult embarrassed Carol and always brought back that bleak, hopeless feeling.

Although Carol's father was ultimately successful in his life as an executive, times were tough when Carol was growing up.

Money was extremely tight. Very little was spent on the children. The only way Carol could have anything for herself was to work hard at odd jobs and babysitting. She hoarded her money carefully. Her sisters and brother made fun of her, borrowed from her, and, in a couple of cases, stole from her. Her father praised her for being hardworking and conservative with money. She also did well in school and worked hard to be the perfect kid, which also brought more approval from Dad.

Carol's extreme sense of responsibility and perfectionism brought an additional benefit. Her father was an alcoholic and when he drank, became violent. Her sisters and brother often caught the brunt of his anger because they often caused trouble. Carol lived a different rule: Make no mistakes and act as you are expected to act. Carol escaped brutal beatings by living this way. She was a sharp counterpoint to her siblings, all of whom eventually had serious alcohol and drug problems. Two of her sisters were victims of domestic abuse, and her brother served eighteen months in prison for embezzlement.

Carol could remember her sisters' promiscuity in high school. On a couple of occasions one of her brother's boyfriends had sex with each of her sisters all in one afternoon. She was sure her brother had participated in one of these events, but she did not want to know. Her mother did not help. She was more like a buddy to the kids, often siding with them against their father. She was keenly interested in what the kids were doing sexually and was always talking about it. They would frequently talk about "boobs"—who had them, who did not, who showed them, and who did not. She flirted outrageously with the girls' boyfriends, making suggestive comments. Carol could remember her mom in a low-cut dress bending over and asking the boys how they liked the view. Everyone laughed. Feeling deeply ashamed, Carol went to her room.

Carol connected sex with the dysfunction and violence of her family. Filled with terror and shame, she used strategies

11

that worked: Be the good, perfect person who did not make mistakes and who acted the role expected of her. She also believed to her core that if she were sexual, she would be like her family. With Chet she was in a bind: To act the role of what was expected of her as a wife would keep her safe, but it also meant she had to be sexual, which filled her with feelings of terror, shame, and anger. She opted for safety.

With bitter tears Carol shared her story with Chet and their therapist. When it came to the point of revealing her dishonesty, she could hardly say she was sorry because of her heartfelt sobs. Yet there was also relief in finally telling her secret. Everyone in the room knew that the truth had shifted reality. Chet and Carol's relationship would never be the same. There was no way to go back once the truth was out.

Miriam, the therapist, gently guided Carol out of the bind she was in. First, Miriam observed that we are so used to our own history, we do not see it as remarkable or out of the ordinary, whereas others might see it as horrendous. Further, we tend to minimize that which we feel shameful about. In a culture such as ours that suffers tremendous shame about sex, we tend to be even less candid about that particular issue. Finally, Miriam noted that using courtship as a path out of pain and suffering is often delusional and deceptive. Sex is fundamental to our lives and it therefore becomes a mirror of our larger issues.

Sex Is Fundamental

As a therapist who has counseled thousands of couples, families, and individuals, I have seen the same lesson emerge over and over again: Sex seems to be the area of life that most deeply touches our personal issues. Whatever problems we face in life sooner or later impact our sexuality. If we are chronically angry, the anger will eventually become sexualized. If we cannot tolerate closeness, we will fail at sexual intimacy. If we need to be in control, passion will elude us. If we have experienced trauma, we may repeat it compulsively through how we express our sexuality. If we are perfectionistic, sexual response will elude us. And, if we are so overextended and driven that all of our important relationships are abbreviated, sex will seem brief and overrated.

To put it in another way, we can hide with sex, we can hide from sex, but we cannot be fully ourselves sexually and hide. Our sexual behavior is a core expression of who we are. The fact that "there is no magic switch" will appear throughout this book. We do not change fundamental personality traits or beliefs when we become sexual. Issues that we have in general, we will also have sexually. No technique or method will change that.

For Chet and Carol there was no mystery about how they got together. When they first started therapy, the apparent problem was that Chet was seeing prostitutes and had had an affair. With time it became clear that his real problem was sexual addiction. Like compulsive gamblers or alcoholics, sex addicts deal with their stress and anxiety by having sex. Often, the more dangerous or somehow illicit the sex is, the more compelling it will be. Most sex addicts have a history of addictions in their families and a history of some form of child abuse. In most cases, they have other compulsions and addictions as well. Chet was also a compulsive spender, which is typical of those involved compulsively with prostitutes. In fact, Miriam pointed out to Carol that her father probably was a sex addict as well, given that her parents had divorced as his extramarital affairs and prostitution use made the marriage untenable. She suggested that part of Chet and Carol's attraction for each other was, in fact, that they came from the same type of family. Carol protested that she had not been sexually abused in the way that Chet had been. Not so, responded her therapist: "That awful feeling you had with your father when it came to sex was his objectifying you and the arousal it provided for him. He did not have to touch you for abuse to have its impact."

Carol was learning that she was a sexual anorexic. Like a food anorexic, she was terrified of her own sexual appetite. She relied on her disciplined and self-sacrificing habits to keep her life in tight control. She compulsively saved as a way to feel safer, which brought her into sharp conflict with Chet and his out-of-control spending. Like many sexual anorexics, she acted sexual as a way to preserve safety and harmony. But she despised her sexuality.

When Chet and Carol met, she was attracted to his sexual ease and his spontaneity with money. She wanted to have fun in her life. Chet similarly hoped that Carol's discipline and frugality would help him in what he already knew to be a problem. In fact, he hoped that sex with Carol would help him to stop the sexual behavior he detested in himself. In fact, both partners hated their sexuality. And nothing was as it seemed.

Sex in the Extremes

In order to get past appearances and gain clarity about sex, we have to start with the basics. First, people can be amazingly diverse in how they are sexual. Every now and then I think I have heard of everything a person can do sexually. Then I meet someone and find myself saying, "I didn't know you could do that." Invariably, I then meet others who do that also. There is tremendous diversity in sexual expression. When pioneering American sexologist Alfred Kinsey was asked what is abnormal, he responded, "Anything you cannot do!"

Second, people also vary in how much sexual experience they have in their lives. Some people have more and some less. Figure 1.1 on page 10 uses a statistician's normal curve to visualize degrees of sexual experience. Most people, whether they tend toward the "more" or toward the "less," fall under the main part of the curve. Some people fall further to the right. That does not mean they are pathological. It may mean they took more risks or had more opportunity. It might be that their sex lives were extremely fulfilling. On the extreme right of the curve, however, is a group of people for whom sexuality has become pathological. Beyond having more sexual experience than others, they have difficulty stopping their sexual behavior. Sex therapists call them "sex addicts," and they have very definite characteristics:

- They have a pattern of out-of-control sexual behavior.
- They continue in that pattern even though it is destroying their lives.
- They will often pursue dangerous or high-risk sex.
- They are sexual even when they do not intend to be.
- They have serious life consequences because of their sexual behavior.
- Their sexual behavior affects their work, hobbies, friends, and families.
- They use sex to help them control their moods and manage stress and anxiety.
- They obsess about sexual things so much that it interferes with normal living.
- They may have periods when they extinguish all sexual behavior and become sex aversive.

Sexual addiction is not about moral weakness or lack of character. In fact, the harder addicts try to change their behavior the worse it gets. Like all addicts, they have an addiction that is about attempting to manage emotional pain.[2]

On the other end of the curve are people whose sexual experience may be sharply curtailed. They may not have had much opportunity. Or maybe they lived in a community or family that had extremely restrictive rules about sexual behavior. Or maybe by personality and experience, they were extremely shy and introverted which limited their ability to initiate sexual contact. Or maybe something organic such as diabetes or high blood pressure limited their ability to be sexual. Conditions like alcoholism or the use of antidepressants can affect sexual desire. Similarly, dysfunctional relationships will dampen sexual ardor. People can also be inhibited because of misinformation, lack of information, previous bad experiences, or all the above.

Figure 1.1

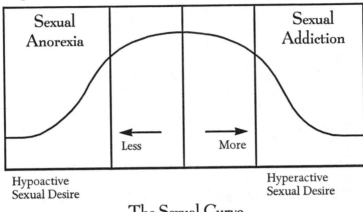

The Sexual Curve

On the extreme left of the curve, however, not being sexual because of a fundamental terror of one's sexuality and a deeply felt hatred for one's sexual feelings is pathological. Sometimes such individuals are sexual when they do not want to be, as in Carol's case. More often they become a "closed system," resisting or avoiding anything connected with sex. Sex becomes the enemy. Therapists call them "sexual anorexics" and they, too, have definite common characteristics:

- They have a pattern of resistance to anything sexual.
- They continue that pattern even though they know it is self-destructive.
- They will go to extremes to avoid sexual contact or attention, including self-mutilation, distortions of body appearance or apparel, and aversive behavior.

- They have rigid, judgmental attitudes toward their own sexuality and the sexuality of others.
- Their resistance and aversion to things sexual help to manage anxiety and to avoid deeper, more painful life issues.
- They have extreme shame and self-loathing about sexual experiences, their bodies, and sexual attributes.
- Their sexual aversion affects their work, hobbies, friends, and families.
- They obsess about sex so much that it interferes with normal living.
- They may have episodes of sexual bingeing or periods of sexual compulsivity.

Again, sexual anorexia is not about character. Sexual anorexics do not wish for the torment of obsession and the demands of rigid control. They recognize that the satisfaction and safety they feel in giving in to their obsession is but temporary. Despite this, the obsession not only does not go away, it somehow feeds on itself.

In many ways, looking at sexual anorexia is like looking at the negative of a black-and-white photograph. All the shades of light and dark are reversed. Addiction and anorexia are shades of the same obsession. A way to understand that is to return to the analogy of the normal curve—only this time think of healthy eating and eating disorders. First, the food people eat can be extraordinarily diverse. The types of food and different methods of preparation make food a wonderful journey of discovery. Second, there exists tremendous diversity in patterns of eating. Some people make eating a top priority and some do not. For some people, eating is such a priority they become compulsive overeaters. They use the soothing, comforting experience of eating to help manage their anxiety, stress, and pain. The result can be extreme obesity and death. When food is used to self-destructive excess, it is addictive.[3]

Moving toward the other end of the curve are people who

eat less food for all the reasons we can imagine: scarcity, metabolism, culture, family, and religion. Yet on the far end is a group of people whose food priority is so low that they are starving themselves. They are terrified of food and obsessed with thinness. This is anorexia nervosa. It can also be highly addictive and deadly. Hans Heubner, an expert on eating disorders, describes anorexia as "having all the characteristics of drug addiction."[4]

One of the more fascinating patterns in eating disorders is how a compulsive overeater will flip from one end of the curve to the other and become a compulsive dieter. Both the anorexic and the overeater have an obsession with food, which is what connects the family of eating disorders. Some go to both extremes out of the same obsession. They will binge-eat as a way to soothe themselves and then they will purge themselves by vomiting or using diuretics and laxatives. This binge-purge phenomenon, or bulimia, is the destructive combination of both extremes.

Sexual bulimics exist as well. These people binge sexually and then plunge into terrible sexual self-hatred. Once we understand this, we begin to read newspaper headlines differently. Picture a well-known clergyman who for years leads a national campaign against pornography. He holds large fund-raising rallies asking tens of thousands of people to kneel and pray with him that the scourge of pornography be lifted from the land. Then the preacher himself gets arrested for the production and distribution of child pornography. Stunned followers and colleagues ask how this could be. Simple. In his private life, he was bingeing and in his public life he was purging. Like the addict, the sexual bulimic has a tremendous capacity to compartmentalize. Just think of clergy in recent years who preached against pornography, prostitution, infidelity, or sexual exploitation and then created huge scandals because of their sexual behavior. In fact, I have many colleagues who take the position that the more extreme, judgmental, and negative religious preachers become, the more suspect they are of having a dark, secret life. The irony of this, as we will see later in this book, is that healthy, successful sex and a well-developed spiritual life are inextricably linked.

Over the years, therapists have treated thousands of sex addicts. Once we started keeping track of the binge-purge phenomenon in our program admissions, we found that 72 percent of sex addicts could more accurately be designated as sexual bulimics. Even those sex addicts whose sexual compulsivity is constant report moments of unbearable despair, for which the only solution is to act out even more. The constant is profound sexual self-hatred.

Understanding Sexual Deprivation

For a long time, addiction specialists have used the word *addiction* to describe persons who compulsively "act out" sexually. More recently, they have incorporated *sexual anorexic* and *sexual bulimic* into their lexicon as understanding of the illness expands. In part, this terminology reflects the parallels and the high degree of interactivity between the eating disorders and the sexual impulse disorders. It also reflects the reality, recognized by clinicians, that a family of addictive disorders exists that includes alcoholism, drug addiction, gambling, sex addiction, and compulsive spending, *as well as* compulsive deprivations such as anorexia nervosa, sexual anorexia, compulsive saving and hoarding, and some phobic responses. The most important new insight of all is that the compulsive deprivation of one substance or behavior is frequently used to balance off the excess of another—in the same person.

Specialists in sexual medicine have long recognized these extremes as well. To return to Figure 1.1, they have described sex addicts as located on the "hyperactive" sexual end of the continuum and anorexics as located on the "hypoactive" sexual end of the continuum. The most severe cases on the hyposexual end are described as "sexual aversion disorder." These specialists also note the parallels between and coexistence of the eating disorders. Although specialists agree that these extremes exist, there is some debate about whether to describe the extremes in addiction terms or as aspects of obsessive compulsive disorder. It should be noted that the current *Diagnostic and Statistical Manual of Mental Disorders* of the American Psychiatric Association clearly states that sexual compulsion is not to be confused with obsessive compulsive disorder, an anxiety disorder that involves the compulsive need to repeat certain physical or mental behaviors.[5] Those who write about addiction have long argued that compulsion is basic to the addictive process. In short, understanding of the problem has outstripped the categories by which to describe it. The field of sexual medicine is experiencing a paradigm shift, which means that as therapists learn more, old ideas give way to new, more expanded models to make sense out of an expanded reality.[6]

I have chosen to use the words *sexual anorexia* because they are easily understood by the people who have the problem. They also create access to the "sexual anorexia" groups that already exist within Twelve Step fellowships such as Sex and Love Addicts Anonymous, Sexaholics Anonymous, Sex Addicts Anonymous, and Sexual Compulsives Anonymous that have been so helpful to so many. On a conceptual basis, describing the problem as *sexual anorexia* facilitates one of the primary ideas of this book: sexual anorexia is embedded in a series of dynamics between excessive behavior and deprivation behavior. To focus simply on the sexual is to miss the more fundamental rhythms that make recovery so elusive. Finally, because it identifies the condition as an illness, *sexual anorexia* connotes the very real possibilities of change to sexual fulfillment.

Much has already been written about sex addicts and those who sexually binge. Not much has been written for the sexually anorexic. To be sure, there is a wealth of books about how to be sexual. Many of these, however, focus on techniques and attitudes. Also, there exists an even greater number of books on relationships and intimacy. These often do not fit the reality of someone living in the extremes. Neither category deals with the most fundamental aspect of recovery from any addiction or compulsion: the essential loss of self that comes with living in the extremes. The sex addict who switches into the anorexic side, for example, only knows the terror of not wanting to return to the nightmare of loss of control. Trauma survivors who binge-eat to cope with life and their terror of sexual contact only know what keeps them safe, not what helps them to be human. So we are on a different journey.

According to a recent large survey, one in five Americans is not interested in sex. If this is correct, that would involve over forty million adults.[7] People might ask, "If I do not have sex, does that make me sexually anorexic?" No. It means many factors—biology, personal development, relationships—can diminish sexual desire. This is why problems with sexual desire are the number one issue sex therapists deal with. However, sexual anorexics do have a definite profile that separates them from the larger population of those having difficulty being sexual:

- They are often extremely competent people who are committed to doing things very well and have a fear of making mistakes and being human.
- They tend to be judgmental of others and themselves when things do not measure up to their superhuman standards.
- They have a history of sexual exploitation or sexual rejection, either perceived or real—or both.
- They have a deep-seated sexual terror because of their history of abuse and rejection.
- They have a sexual self-hatred that dominates their lives.
- They come from families with a history of addictions, and they tend to extreme or addictive behavior themselves.
- They use rigidity as a defense to feeling out of control.
- They often have secrets and insane loyalties of which they may not be consciously aware.

- They are often caught in double binds because of those secrets and insane loyalties.
- They can be extremely creative but feel constrained and unproductive with no sense of why they feel that way.
- They have been deeply influenced by a cultural, family, or social message that sex in some way is negative.

The fact that sexual anorexics are different from the larger population of those who are not very sexual does not diminish very real problems for all of us. We live in a culture that does not support sexual development. Worse, it does much to harm our sexuality. Also, we are living in a time of extraordinary, profound change in sexual mores, beliefs, and practices. Before we can understand compulsive sexual deprivation, we must first outline these bigger issues.

The Sex-Negative Culture

Sex is problematic in our culture. Sexual liberation in the 1960s and 1970s was welcomed as an antidote to the prudish, sex-negative messages of the nineteenth century. Myriad examples from the Victorian era exist documenting the extreme discomfort with sexual issues during those times. The fashion of putting skirts on piano legs because they might prove suggestive is an example of the cultural extremes of that epoch. In some ways cultural dynamics parallel some of the personal dynamics we described under the curve in figure 1.1. The counterpoint to the excessive, and often religiously based, fear of things sexual for the Victorians is that childhood sexual abuse and prostitution use surged as well in that century.[8]

With Sigmund Freud in the early part of this century, a movement started toward a deeper acknowledgment of the importance of sex in our lives. The growing understanding of mental health, the significance of the women's movement, and the incredible impact of the communications industry have combined to break down barriers to sexual understanding. Yet, we are hardly living in a culture of sexual comfort. In fact, as we look around in North America there are signs of deep sexual discontent:

- The divorce rate in recent years has included 50 percent of new marriages.
- Over half of all women will experience sexual assault at some time in their lives.
- Only one in twenty sexual assaults is reported.
- Over one million women are victims of domestic physical violence annually.
- Five hundred thousand adolescents work as prostitutes every year.
- Forty-two percent of women who are murdered knew their attackers well.
- One in ten college students admits to date rape.[9]

Despite our progress in talking about sexual issues, we can hardly say we live in a culture that is positive toward sex. The sexual terrain of our times is filled with fear, uncertainty, and reactivity.

An example is the research into child abuse. In the 1980s, research on posttraumatic stress disorder in Vietnam veterans was regarded as important, noble, and useful. When the same researchers looked at the same problem in children who had been sexually abused, a tremendous controversy ensued—a controversy that persists to this day. There were those who disputed the extent and severity of the sexual abuse that had been uncovered. Similarly, addiction medicine research into gambling and eating disorders generated normal academic and clinical controversies. But describing people as addicted who had the identical symptoms as a result of sexual behaviors generated tremendous controversy. We could accept gambling as an addiction but not sex. Thus, while we have made extraordinary progress, it was not without turmoil, and we clearly have a considerable way to go toward becoming a sex-positive culture.

Another example of our sex-negative culture is sex education in the schools. Some parents mobilize to prevent their children from learning the basics about sexuality. Although some of these parents insist that sex education is a matter for the home, their children frequently report a no-talk rule in their homes regarding sex. Again, we are making progress, but experts report a growing backlash against sex education. The backlash represents a deep-seated distrust of things sexual.

If anthropologists from another species were to do an ethnographic study of our culture, they would be struck by the themes that seem to emerge. These themes distort and distress our sexual lives.

Sex as Manipulation

Women's and men's magazines that feature articles on how to get the upper hand in a relationship and how to get our needs met in the sexual combat zone sell well on newsstands. A steady stream of best-sellers offers advice on the battle between the sexes. The extraordinary success of books like *Men Are from Mars, Women Are from Venus* by John Gray or *The Rules* by Ellen Fein and Sherrie Schneider or *The Code* by Nate Penn and Lawrence Larose simply reflects the tremendous confusion people feel about sexuality and their desire to resolve it. Courtship and romance, however, are not going to be enhanced by outmaneuvering the object of our affections.

Sex as Trauma

Traumatic sex is one of the norms of our culture. The examples are all around us, in our movies, television shows, in the tabloids, and splashed across the headlines and lead stories of mainstream media. Blockbuster movies like *Pulp Fiction*, *The Piano*, *Fatal Attraction*, and *Disclosure* are part of a stream of stories that fuse sex with violence, exploitation, and danger. Our news media obsess about stories of a similar mix: the bizarre, sexual murder of a child beauty pageant queen; the Nobel laureate arrested for child molestation; the errant bishop whose sexual encounters with children prompted him to commit suicide rather than deal with his accusers. We are obsessed with the serial lust murderer whether it be the real story of a Jeffrey Dahmer or the fictitious story of a Hannibal Lechter in *Silence of the Lambs*.

We have been obsessed with the sexual life of the British Royal Family and the antics of our presidents (JFK and Marilyn Monroe, President Clinton's struggle with Paula Jones—or the portrayals of the "fictional" presidents in *Primary Colors* and *Absolute Power*). The seemingly endless list of political figures— Justice Clarence Thomas, Senator Robert Packwood, Senator Gary Hart, and presidential advisor Dick Morris—who have been in trouble sexually results in a distrust of political leadership.

Nor have churches been exempt. The televangelists alone have had followers shaking their heads. Current estimates are that up to 6 percent of Catholic priests have been sexually involved with children, and that less than 2 percent actually maintain celibacy over the course of a career. 28 percent are reportedly in ongoing heterosexual relationships and 13 percent are in gay relationships. Catholics are traumatized by the fact that over a billion dollars have been spent in court settlements, and many parents no longer trust priests with their children.[10] Similar stories can be told for Protestant denominations, as well as variations of Judaism. Studies of Protestant clergy indicate that up to 23 percent of married clergy have affairs with parishioners.[11] In the mid-1990s, the West Coast reeled with stories of child abuse by rabbis. I believe that religion in America has been fundamentally altered by the sexual misconduct of clergy who have exploited their positions of pastoral care.

Our entertainment, our political leaders, and our religious

leadership continue to provide examples of sexuality coupled with violence, exploitation, and deception. We are like the child in the family who is not abused. While the abuse may not have happened to us directly, such traumatic occurrences undermine our feelings of safety and trust. The result is a climate that mirrors the fearful terrors that sexual anorexics already have.

Sex as Marital Failure

A common phenomenon is the cooling of sexual desire after a few years of marriage. Talk shows and other media give much attention to how to rekindle that erotic flame. Much of that advice focuses on techniques of lovemaking and creating interest in one's partner. All of which, however, ignores a more fundamental reality: The structure of work and family in our culture undermines intimacy. A famous family researcher used voice-activated tape recorders to find out what couples really talk about. He found that the average couple spends less than twenty-seven minutes a week in truly intimate conversation. Much of that is because families do not spend much time together.

In earlier times, families worked together, often in extended families. This is the first time in history that society has asked just two people to raise children. Families in the eighteenth century had more child care options than we do now. Today the norm is to spread families across the country, isolated from one another. It is also the norm now for couples to be dual-career families. Dad works in one place, Mom in another, and the children attend different schools. By definition, intimacy is based on shared, common experience. If parents have little help, and little time, there is little shared, common experience. The result is a soaring divorce rate. Therapists and researchers know that family isolation is the core cause of both child abuse and addictive illness. Drug use by adolescents in our culture is soaring. Of the twenty-six most prosperous nations of the world, the United States has the highest rates of violence, murder, and suicide among children. Such tragedy is mostly a result of family stress.[12]

The intimacy that sustains successful sex is undermined by family and cultural stress. In courtship, a couple will make time together a priority, and sex works under those circumstances. With marriage, the culture starts to cut into that priority, however, and sexuality shifts. Even worse, with men and women working closely together, the priorities become even more confused. If we work side by side with someone fifty to sixty hours a week, we may end up feeling closer to that person than to the one we sleep with. And sexuality follows such closeness. Does getting married mean that sex is over? No. It does mean that for marriage to survive in our culture, we must understand the forces arrayed against marital intimacy. No sexual recovery program can overlook that fact.

Sex as Sleaze

"Sex is dirty, save it for someone you love." I have found over the years that this aphorism never fails to get a laugh from audiences. The humor is in the juxtaposition of two coexisting tenets in our culture. One tenet assumes that to enjoy sex a person has to walk the seamy side of life. Prostitution, massage parlors, strip joints, affairs, unwed mothers, out-of-control drinking, and backseat sex come to mind. Unless sex is illicit, it will not be good. In recent years, the use of sex to sell goods is a variation of the "sleaze factor" in the sense that sex becomes part of sales manipulation or corporate exploitation.

The other tenet is that sex belongs as part of a committed relationship, which connotes high values, but low passion. Honor and virtue do not seem to combine well with deep desire. Men are presented with a choice of the Madonna or the whore. The real man chooses both but will have to be dishonest about it. Women are presented with a double standard: Men can do things women cannot. Women are put in the role of guardians of morality and are therefore failures as women if they "succumb" to their sexual natures. Children, adolescents, and the elderly are not supposed to have any sexual feelings at all.

Religious traditions have, in fact, been part of this split way of understanding sexuality. The ideas of sex as sin outside of marriage and sex as duty inside of marriage have gone far to undermine the acceptance of sexual pleasure as normal or healthy. Official church doctrine or policy has certainly not supported sexual exploitation and the laity have been stunned by revelations of sexual abuse by church leaders. The result is a crisis within churches and synagogues that calls them to reexamine the sexual assumptions behind doctrines and customs. As mentioned earlier, the irony is that sexual transformation and spiritual renewal probably cannot occur separately.

Both stereotypes of sexual expression (sin and duty) have begun to weaken with the changes in sexual thinking of recent decades. Yet most adults reading this book know these sexual biases well and have been affected by them. What is missing is the idea and practice of fundamental equality and mutual respect between the sexes as well as permission for a deep acceptance for the fact that, as discussed earlier, *sex is fundamental*—to both sexes and to all ages. People working to reclaim their sexuality need to understand that they are doing this task within the context of an era of extraordinary, culture-wide change in our sexual perspectives.

Sex as Oppression

An employee of a major United States airline company reported being sexually harassed at work. She asked her supervisors for help, but nothing meaningful happened. She filed an official complaint, but again nothing was done. Not long after taking that action, she was found murdered in the trunk of her car. Although employees accused in the harassment complaint were suspected, the corporation maintained it had no responsibility for what happened. But I believe they do. I think we all do. Whenever we participate in sexual prejudices that support exploitation, whether it be through compliance, denial, or inaction, we are guilty.

Sexual oppression respects neither sexual orientation nor gender. We might use the American armed services as a cultural mirror on sexual issues. "Don't Ask, Don't Tell," the official military attitude toward gay and lesbian recruits, reflects an uneasy and a contradictory compromise regarding acceptance of sexual diversity in our country. The reality of this policy is that homosexuality is fine as long as we all pretend it doesn't exist; which is, of course, another way of saying it's not all right. Similarly, women now can fight side by side with men in the armed forces. Yet the Pentagon reports over a billion dollars have been spent dealing with sexual harassment settlements and claims. The U.S. Navy Tailhook scandal, the brutal hazing of the first female cadets at the Citadel, the discharge against their will of homosexual service members who refuse to deny who they are—these incidents become icons, markers on the sexual battlefield. In World War I opposing armies fought over the same few miles of land in Flanders for years before there was resolution. The fight against prejudice based on sexual orientation or gender seems to also be an interminable struggle. Just because something has been made a legal reality does not make it real in people's lives, a fact those who have long fought against racial prejudice know too well.

Few stories encapsulate the dark side of our culture as well as the O. J. Simpson saga played out on national television in the mid-1990s. It had all the key elements of tabloid fascination: race, domestic violence, great wealth, sexual excess, substance abuse, double murder, and vulnerable children. Few stories encapsulate the dark side of our culture as the tragedy of that double homicide and its legal aftermath. Only one, the Clarence Thomas/Anita Hill battle for credibility over issues of alleged sexual harassment, presented to the public via nationally televised Congressional hearings, has come close in national obsession—precisely because it has many of the same elements. Whether we saw O. J. as the victim of the white establishment or Nicole Brown Simpson as the victim of an out-of-control patriarchy, there exists a piece of all of us in the story. Whether you see Clarence Thomas as the victim of a below-the-belt ideological attack or as someone who abused his power in the workplace in order to attempt to blackmail someone into giving him sexual favors, there is little question that it is reflective of a battle that is played out in workplaces across the nation.

For the sexual anorexic as well as for the sex addict, these dark themes create a toxic sexual environment that makes sex very problematic. Both extremes—the sexual anorexic and the addict—struggle with a deep-seated terror of their own sexuality. In a culture in which sex is about manipulation, or about trauma, or about sleaze, or about marital failure, or about oppression, the terror has much to draw on. Recovery from compulsive sexual disorders can only proceed with a realistic appreciation of the formidable cultural forces arrayed against it.

Yet, there is a greater significance to all this. All these issues are symptomatic of a time of extraordinary social change, the core of which is sexual. There is coming a paradigm shift—or expansion of our understanding—of a significance parallel to the changes that accompanied the writing of the Magna Charta or the advent of Galileo's telescope. As with all changes of this magnitude, it is accompanied by struggle and conflict. We must not get lost in the turmoil, however, for embedded in the new paradigm is a new model for sexual well-being. Recovery from substance or behavior addiction or compulsion can draw from and contribute to this emerging consciousness.

Toward a New Paradigm

The change has been long coming. Social historians Philippe Aries and Georges Duby in their massive multivolume series, *A History of Private Life*, trace the evolution of Western culture from the time of ancient Greece and Rome to the dawn of modern times. Their painstaking collection of data about family, marriage, sexuality, and lifestyle is not about kings, empires, wars, or governments. Rather, it is a series of portraits about how ordinary people lived their lives. Basically, it is the story of movement from corporate reality to individual reality. In earlier times, people's intimate life was defined by their guild, family, clan, or church. There were few choices about intimacy they could make themselves. Marriages were arranged since they were about alliances and not individual fulfillment. Privacy and sexual fulfillment were actually foreign concepts until relatively modern times. In the scale of centuries, the empowerment of the individual to be all that she or he can be is a relatively recent notion. With individualism came a revolution in sexual expression as important as the rise of capitalism or modern science. The famous historian Peter Gay describes this shift as literally "the education of the senses."[13]

Parallel with individual awareness and sexual expression came individual responsibility. Historians who study the abuse of children over time note that as self-awareness expanded so did prohibitions against the sexual exploitation and physical abuse of children. In many of the ancient city-states, a father had the right to terminate the life of a child. Thus, a valley outside of the city of Carthage was found to contain 20,000 urns filled with the bones of infants who had been sacrificed in religious ritual. The sexual abuse of children was a common part of the social fabric of the time. Authors from Plato to Plutarch described it.[14]

By the Middles Ages it was a sin to have sex with a child. If an adult were guilty of such a sin, one remedy was to declare the child a witch. The child thus became an offender who "beguiled" the adult with the power of the Evil One.

Understanding this process puts a new light on the burning of witches. A Catholic bishop in Wurttemberg in the seventeenth century writes, for example, of his sadness at having presided over the burning of three hundred young girls that year and of his wonder if the church were making a mistake.[15]

By the nineteenth century, society had given up burning witches. Yet the sexual exploitation of children continued. In late-nineteenth-century Britain, for example, men who raped young girls were excused because they did it to cure venereal disease. There was a widely held belief that children would take "poisons" out of the body. In fact, leprosy, venereal disease, depression, and impotence were part of a wide range of maladies believed cured by having sex with the young. An English medical text of the time reads, "Breaking a maiden's seal is one of the best antidotes for one's ills. Cudgeling her unceasingly, until she swoons away, is a mighty remedy for man's depression. It cures all impotence."

We have come a long way since those days. Yet only in the last thirty years have we taken a meaningful public stand against child abuse. One of the leading experts on the history of child abuse, Lloyd DeMause, writes of the significance of this moment in our cultural evolution:

> A society's childrearing practices are not just one item in a list of cultural traits, but—because all other traits must be passed down from generation to generation through the narrow funnel of childhood—actually makes childrearing the very basis for the transmission and development of all other cultural traits, placing definite limits on what can be achieved in the material spheres of history. Regardless of the changes in the environment, it is only when real progress in childrearing occurs that societies begin to progress and move in unpredictable new directions that are more adaptive.[16]

Essentially, child development scholars see this time as pivotal in the evolution of our species, especially sexually.

Few have explored this massive change in our sexuality with more understanding than Riane Eisler in her landmark books *The Chalice and the Blade* and *Sacred Pleasure*. Eisler reviewed and synthesized findings in archeology and anthropology from the 1950s through the 1980s. She found cultures who were very successful at peace but who were largely unknown to the public. Some of these cultures endured many centuries without war. They were sophisticated in science, art, theology, and economics. Characteristics they had in common were

- a collaborative, democratic culture that put a high emphasis on partnership, affiliation, and each individual's contribution
- an essential equality between men and women with real roles of power and authority for both and with permission for each to take sexual initiative with no advantage over the other
- an essential aversion to rigidity, abuse of power, and exploitive competition
- a commitment to respectful, passionate but nonexploitive sexuality that precluded the abuse of children

Eisler traces the history of how a patriarchal, competitive, and exploitive culture replaced earlier partnership societies and not only became the norm, but also rewrote history in its own dominator-model image.

The world is shrinking. What happens in the Gulf of Aqaba and Hong Kong significantly affects matters in your town—wherever you live. A competitive, exploitive ethic, left to run rampant in the world, will eventually destroy it. Eisler makes the case that if we want to change, it will have to start with how men and women treat each other sexually and how we raise our children. In the age of CNN and the Internet, the world is a witness to how the postindustrial society finally comes to grips with fundamental sexual issues.

Some say the coming paradigm change will be extraordinary. Denise Breton and Christopher Largent describe this watershed in their very important book, *The Paradigm Conspiracy: How Our Systems of Government, Church, School, and Culture Violate Our Human Potential.* They say the new paradigm is emerging on many fronts: environmentalism, progress in mental health, the men's and women's movements, the reassertion of the values of Native American and other indigenous peoples, and the technology that breaks down cultural walls. We are moving to interconnectedness at blinding speed. They write:

> [Connectedness is] our most basic need, from which all other needs grow. Born in a connected universe, our foremost need is to connect—with ourselves and those around us; with the environment that includes the food chain and life-support systems; with family, educational, economic, and political systems; with ideas and human evolution; with meaning and purpose. Experiencing our connectedness to its fullest is what being alive in a connected universe means.
>
> Our need to experience our connectedness—and to act in ways that affirm it—doesn't mean we're inherently selfish or criminal. It simply shows that we understand our existence to be woven into expanding patterns, without which we cannot exist. Far from making us behave selfishly, cultivating an awareness of our connected existence affirms us as an integral part of larger tapestries.[17]

Key to this process is a common set of principles to govern our relationships. They emerge from the confederation principles of the Iroquois and the Twelve Steps of the various anonymous fellowships. They are the same ones identified by Eisler in the successful societies: self-responsibility, permission to grow, sexual equality and joy, collaboration and partnership, and a fundamental respect for the earth, children, and each other.

The premises of this book are simple. People at each end of the sexual continuum have been damaged. Indeed, all of us have. The forces of the past and the chaos of the present have left little room to escape. Out of the sexual extremes of anorexia and addiction, however, have come voices that articulate where the damage really lies. Embedded in the recovery way of life are principles of sexual health—which for the most part have not been articulated, let alone celebrated. The implications for you, dear reader, are several:

- that you are not alone in the pain you have experienced, and that your hurt is real
- that there is a better way to peace within our sexual lives
- that your courage to proceed on this journey helps not only you but also all of us who want healing on this planet
- that we in this generation are addressing not only the needs of children now and in the future, but also the children within ourselves

To begin, we must start with understanding sex as deprivation.

SEX AS DEPRIVATION

Yen-yang asked Chao-chou, "What if I have
nothing with me?"
Chao-chou said, "Throw it away!"
Yen-yang said, "If I have nothing with me,
what can I throw away?"
Chao-chou said, "In that case, keep
holding it."[1]

—Hung-chih Cheng-chueh

"I'M SEXUALLY ANOREXIC," said Shannon. "I would not feel sexual and I wanted to be. And it was real painful. The best way to describe it is that it was like this huge concrete wall. I would think that I wanted to be sexual because I had the feelings, but it simply would be too close. It felt like too much and this huge wall of resistance would be in front of me," she continued. Shannon then looked at me with tears brimming in her eyes and said, "My mind would think of the 2,953 reasons why I shouldn't be sexual or why not at that moment or that time of day or whatever. . . . It became this real painful battle." She collected herself, took a deep breath, and concluded, "At the time I thought that 'healthy sexuality'—whatever that was—simply would not be powerful enough to pull me through whatever that concrete barrier was."

To look at Shannon and her husband, Ben, we would not guess they had been through such turmoil. To the external world they look like two very successful, attractive professional people in their late forties. They are prompt, efficient, and responsible. They also are good parents with kids in good schools. There is not the slightest clue as to the painful struggle the two of them endured. Actually, this is the second marriage for both Ben and Shannon. Ben lost his first marriage because of his alcoholism. Getting remarried was scary for him because he had been sexual only when he was using or "wasted," as he put it.

Shannon lost her first marriage because of her sexual anorexia. She described it this way, "I did not want to be sexual so it was a power struggle, and I got shamed a lot, so I went through years of just defending myself. And in the long run, he left because I was not sexual enough. He was very clear about that."

Now Shannon and Ben are married again and have two children, and sex is safe and rewarding. Years of recovery and therapy have made a difference. I asked them to talk with me about what life was like before therapy and what it was like now. Both partners agreed that now what happened internally matched what showed in the outside world. "What you see is what you get," Shannon explained. The old way was a world of secrecy, deception, and control. For Shannon it was about hiding her terror of sex; for Ben it was about anesthetizing his pain and fear.

Many anorexics project a world of being under control. In fact, the external world of the anorexic is often filled with compliance and, ironically, with an effort to meet everyone else's needs. Anorexics tend to be perfectionistic and spend a great deal of energy attempting to cover all the bases. Much energy goes into looking good and shoring up any holes that may appear in that image. This is where the pain starts, in the tremendous distance between idealistic expectations and actual performance. With sex, the distance between the fantasy of what the anorexic thinks sex should be like and the internal reality is a constant source of pain. So how can someone so focused on meeting the needs of others be so committed to not responding to sexual needs? To understand that, we have to enter the interior world of the sexual anorexic.

The Interior World of the Anorexic

Sexual anorexia usually starts with abandonment or betrayal. Sexual abuse would do it. But so would a profound rejection by a loved one—or exploitation by a loved one. Whatever the initial trauma, the pain was so great that the anorexic made a fundamental, unconscious commitment: Never combine intimacy and sexuality. To do so would resurrect the pain of the trauma and make oneself vulnerable to more trauma. The solution is control, and doing things for other people is one way to control them since they will, in time, grow to depend on the anorexic. Perfectionism is another strategy for control. Making sure every part of one's external life is in order is a way to protect oneself from surprises, from the unknown. Having things in order also protects against someone finding a flaw and thereby opening the way to further shame and rejection. Yet another way to stay in control is sexual aversion; no one can, after all, force the anorexic to have an orgasm.

Control

An unexpected outcome of excessive giving as a form of control is that the giver becomes depleted. There is an essential loss of the sense of who one is. For anorexics in this mode, the denial of sex is not only about sexual safety. Their internal logic dictates, "If I give in and have sex, nothing else is mine." Part of the terror around sex is that they will be used again. But the deeper terror is that if somehow they lose control in the one area in which no one can take control away by force, they cease to be a person. As Shannon put it, "If I give in, then who am I?"

Denial of sex also enables the sexual anorexic to maintain a certain control of the partner. When the anorexic feels out of control, sex can be a way to manipulate another to regain control. And by having control of the partner, the anorexic can also maintain some measure of control over others in the family. If the partner puts pressure on the sexual anorexic to change, that verifies the control the anorexic holds and gives the anorexic even more power. If sexual anorexia is identified, the anorexic can still maintain a certain power by denying the problem. Therapists call this phenomenon "secondary gain," and it is typical of the psychological patterns behind many deprivation behaviors. In food anorexia there is a certain virtue in not overeating, which becomes part of the denial system. With compulsive saving, the person can dismiss the suggestion of a problem by simply asking, "How can being too thrifty be a problem?" (The answer, of course, is when it's part of obsessional self-deprivation.) Similarly, in sexual anorexia some degree of prudish righteousness can enter into the denial arguments, especially if it generates the concern and involvement of the partner and a therapist.

Sexual aversion has several virtues for the anorexic. It keeps things simple and black and white. There is no anxiety-producing confusion or vulnerability. There is a sense of accomplishment about asserting the mind over bodily functions. These "benefits" are consistent with the sexual anorexic's other efforts to control outcomes. Perfectionism and other compulsive deprivations form a pattern of avoidant behaviors. The problem is that the end result for the sexual anorexic is profound self-loathing.

Self-Hatred

Abuse, betrayal, exploitation, and profound rejection—all leave the sexual anorexic with a fundamental conclusion: Somehow he or she is a flawed, defective human being. This conclusion resolves itself into a set of core beliefs that state

- I am basically a bad, unworthy person.
- No one would love me as I am.
- My needs are never going to be met if I have to depend on others.

There is an internal logic here. Once we conclude that we are an unworthy person, we embrace a politics of rejection. We can only assume that other people will reach the same conclusion we have, that they will find us unlovable too. Therefore, others will never meet whatever needs we have because of our unlovable nature. Whatever we ultimately decide to do to take care of ourselves cannot involve reliance on others.

Readers of my book *Out of the Shadows* will quickly recognize these core beliefs as those of the sexual addict and the sexual codependent. Actually, sex addicts and co-sex addicts share these beliefs with sexual anorexics. The difference is how sex addicts and anorexics translate these shame-based core beliefs in their behavior. For sexual anorexics, the involuntary feelings of shame manifest as resistance, the "concrete wall" that Shannon talked about. They do not want to be that way, but that is their interior reality. The consequences of becoming sexual or enjoying sex mean "giving in" to their partner and thereby devaluing themselves. A deep, core resentment of self starts to affect everything in their lives. They are just as "powerless" over their illness as sex addicts and co-addicts, but their focus is different and it comes out differently.

For sexual anorexics, self-hatred often expresses itself as anger. And there is a lot to be angry about. The sexual anorexic is angry at pressure to be sexual by the partner. The anorexic is angry at a culture that seems to create sexual pressure by inserting sex into every part of life. Movies, television, schools, magazines, sales ads, drugstores, newsstands—all become sources of resentment. The anorexic also feels anger at past abuse, betrayal, and rejection. The individual perpetrator, however, becomes lost to the victim in a more generalized anger called "sexualized rage." If the perpetrator was a man, all men receive the rage. Husbands, bosses, employees, friends, and male children may become targets of the anorexic's angry blind prejudice. "All men are like that."

The anorexic also generally feels anger toward the family of origin. If family members were not part of whatever abandonment or abuse occurred, they did not prevent it. The family may have done nothing to facilitate healing, or perhaps failed to teach essential coping skills that may have softened or prevented the pain.

Usually, the rage of sexual anorexia is profoundly passive-aggressive. To not act is a statement of anger that has long gone unrecognized even by professionals. In this case, not acting is paramount since to act (to become sexual) renders the anger meaningless and thereby makes the original betrayal, the first cause of the anger, now somehow acceptable. This goes far beyond inhibited sexual desire and is much more than just being angry with a partner. It represents a fundamental bind that translates to the sexual anorexic as follows: If I am sexual, I am despicable for letting myself down about my deepest wound. If I am not sexual, I will be untrue to my own nature as a sexual being. Either way I will hate myself. But, of the two options, the terror associated with being sexual, with revisiting the original psychosexual trauma, is far, far worse.

Sex as Terror

Behind the anger of the sexual anorexic, then, is a deep and abiding terror. One part of this terror is a powerful, generalized fear of failure. Always doing things well is one strategy for covering up how unworthy the anorexic feels. So on one level, the fear is of disappointing others and not meeting expectations. The deeper fear, however, is the fear of sex. Remember, the primary goal of the sexual anorexic is to find ways to not combine intimacy and sex. When successful sex and intimacy merely serve to open another window to possible betrayal, the aversion to sex becomes the barrier that keeps the private, vulnerable self safe. The terror, as mentioned above, is about reexperiencing the pain. From this dilemma, another core belief emerges: The sexual anorexic believes that "sex is my most terrifying need."

To fully understand how the sexual anorexic reaches this conclusion, we must look further into the making of a sexual anorexic. First, sexual anorexics tend to come from "rigid" families. These families are very controlling. Usually one person is in charge and there is little or no negotiation about the rules. If a family member does not measure up to expectations, punishment is severe, arbitrary, and immediate. A family system is "closed" when the family is extremely resistant to new ideas. It is dangerous in such a family to make a mistake. Perfection is expected. Growing up in this family leaves children with few options. Children can be perfectionistic and try to blend in by adopting the given values of the family or, in an effort to be their own person, resist all demands and become rebellious. Or they may even be both, meaning that on the surface they will appear to adopt the family's values, but secretly they rebel and defy the rules of the family. No matter which option the child chooses, however, there will be fear.

Usually these families tend to be sex negative as well. Sex is treated in a highly moral and condemning fashion. Parents are extremely judgmental and punitive about sexual issues with the children. Yet the children may discover on the part of one or both parents a series of secret sexual behaviors that violate the code preached to the children. In rigid families this is how many offspring learn about having a secret life. At the very least, they learn the lessons taught by little or no affection in a puritanical or sexually anxious family environment.

Anorexics tend also to come from "disengaged" families. This classic dysfunctional family has family members passing each other like the proverbial "ships in the night." They do not have much in common, nor do they share much with each other. Intimacy is very elusive. For children there can be a failure to bond with the parents. They learn not to trust other people and to fear intimacy. As adults they will tend to choose either compulsive avoidant or compulsive addictive behaviors—or some workable combination of both.

The other dysfunctional family system that sometimes leads to sexual anorexia is the "enmeshed" family. The enmeshed family is characterized by too much closeness. Boundaries are broad, vague, or nonexistent. Each family member's business is everyone's business, and there is no sense of emotional privacy or even autonomy. In such families, the child may have difficulty learning how to set boundaries and be a separate person. The end result is that children learn to fear intimacy because their only experience of it was overwhelming. Disengaged or enmeshed—either family system creates children with little trust and tremendous fear of being close.

In addition to these dysfunctional family systems, the sexual anorexic's family of origin usually was marked with substance and/or behavior addictions as well as physical and/or psychological abuse. Shannon spoke of her "raging, alcoholic" father and how she was always attracted to extremely controlling, abusive men. Ben told of his "vicious, sarcastic" mother. For both Shannon and Ben, the opposite-sex parent represented unreliability and outright danger.

For Shannon, a date-rape experience with the son of family friends changed her life forever. In addition to the trauma of the rape itself, the incident represented a double betrayal by her own family. First, no one in her family believed her or took her side because he was "such a wonderful boy." In fact, Shannon's family accused her of misleading him. Second, her family shunned her after the event because she stuck with her story. There was no doubt in her mind as to what had occurred: She had been violated. And yet, she found that the family rules about sex worked against her even when she was the victim. This presents a corollary core belief derived from the dilemma of "sex is my most terrifying need," a belief that serves to magnify the inner terror: "If anything goes wrong during sex, no one will believe me. It will be my fault, no matter what."

Impaired Thinking of the Sexual Anorexic

Based on these core beliefs, distorted thought patterns evolve. Shannon described it this way: "I would get feedback that I was aloof, sort of acting like I was above it all. That was not how I felt inside. And when my first husband told me I was cold and unresponsive, I was surprised. There was no problem here, inside. I did think his demanding sex from me was demeaning." Following years of recovery work, Shannon found she had a very different picture. She now understands that her "being above it all" in terms of Ben's expressions of desire for sex was simply a front. There was a problem, and she was distorting what he was asking for into something ugly and degrading. There was a thought filter at work that justified her distance.

The problem of sexual anorexia begins with denial. "There is no problem," they maintain. Like the food anorexic who denies any feelings of hunger, the sexual anorexic denies sexual thoughts or feelings even in the midst of sexual activity. The anorexic is certain no therapy or help is required. He or she will tend to blame the partner for the tensions surrounding the sexual relationship. The anorexic may view the partner as undisciplined, impulsive, and somewhat immature. In fact, the assumption is that the partner's demands kill the desire in the anorexic. Instead of interpreting sexual overtures as loving and intimate, or as an authentic expression of desire and attraction, the anorexic sees them as suspect, dangerous, threatening. One of the legacies of sexual betrayal is that the survivors can see anything sexual as having an exploitive agenda. It is not surprising, then, that sexual anorexics tend to doubt the sincerity of any sexual advance. No amount of proof to the contrary can persuade them otherwise.

Beyond the anorexic's relationship with his or her partner, all parts of social interaction come under the same scrutiny. The sexual joke of a friend, the sex education program at school, the magazine article on maintaining sexual arousal in marriage, the talk show on prostitution, news about possible sexual indiscretions of actors or politicians—anything that involves sexual content is immediately scrutinized and judged. The interesting exception is sexual misconduct by clergy. The sexual anorexic often will not believe reports of sexual trauma in the church. In part, that disbelief stems from how sex-negative theology has been used to shore up the anorexic's justification of feelings of superiority. To see the body as sinful and without redemption supports the anorexic's rationale for being "above it all" and validates the need for total mastery over sexual feelings. Often, if the church leader is in sexual trouble, the sexual anorexic would rather deny it than admit uncertainty about her or his sexual assumptions. Professionals who work in this area are often stunned by the reaction of congregates who leap to support an errant pastor—even when the evidence is incontrovertible.

Five common thought distortions emerge from the core beliefs of sexual anorexics:

1. Anything erotic is threatening (as opposed to simply human or arousing).
2. Any sexual issue is immediately suspect.
3. Anybody who is sexual is by definition out of control, immoral, base.
4. Any sexual overture or initiation is exploitive or self-serving (as opposed to loving or intimate).
5. Any sexual desire on my partner's part must be balanced by a greater reserve on my part.

For sexual anorexics, an inherent logic evolves from the emotional constriction of the rigid, disengaged, or enmeshed family; the experience of abuse and betrayal; and a sex-negative culture. This tightly woven logic extends beyond the core beliefs into impaired thinking and thought distortion. The result in the interior world of the anorexic is a righteous stance against all things sexual. Figure 2.1 summarizes this interior world.

The Anorexia Cycle

Based on their own internal logic, sexual anorexics enter a self-perpetuating thinking and behavioral cycle that starts with obsessive preoccupation with sexual matters—scanning for potential sexual threat. This obsession leads to distancing strategies that can be widely diverse. Shannon used to take special precautions so as not to be available for sexual overtures from her husband. She claimed to be a "night owl" who would get her "second wind" at night and work to the early morning hours. The real reason for adopting this stance was that this schedule sharply diminished chances of amorous contact. Other distancing strategies used by anorexics include

- dressing in an unattractive or "dowdy" fashion
- dressing in extremely conservative styles that disguise sexuality
- excessive exercise or compulsive dieting to bolster feelings of body mastery
- psychosomatic illnesses that preclude sexual activity
- cutting or mutilating body parts to make oneself unattractive or to symbolize one's sex-negative attitude
- covering or eliminating anything that could possibly stimulate sexual arousal

Shannon said, "I would get into this zone in which nothing could bother me. All avenues were closed. I felt safe, righteous, and in charge. I was proud of myself." This "zone" is also known as sexual aversion: the complete shutting down of

Figure 2.1

The Interior World of the Sexual Anorexic

Maintain Control

- Never combine intimacy and sexuality
- No one can force you to orgasm
- No risk exists to future vulnerability
- No risk of memories of past pain and rejection
- Keep control of partner and family
- Fits other efforts to control outcomes
- Power exists in resistance to change
- Self-esteem feels better when in control
- Sense of accomplishment comes, mind winning over body

Core Beliefs about Self

- I am basically a bad, unworthy person
- No one would love me as I am
- My needs will not be met if I have to rely on others
- Sex is my most terrifying need

Anger for Self and Others

- Core beliefs about being unworthy and unloveable create resentment about self as flawed
- Core belief about being self-sufficient creates resentment toward others
- Anger at partner and culture
- Anger at past perpetrators of betrayal or rejection
- Anger projected on others
- Sexual aversion becomes passive-aggressive response to the survivor's double bind
  - If I am sexual, I let myself down
  - If I am not sexual, I let myself down

Fear of Sex and Intimacy

- Fear of vulnerability
- Fear of sexual success
- Fear of inadequacy and rejection
- Fear of disappointing others and not meeting expectations (terror)
- Fear of reenactment of trauma (terror)
- Fear of pain of past betrayal
- Fear (terror) of sexual needs

Impaired Thinking

- Denial—there is no problem
- Minimization—sex is a lower-order need
- Delusion—I am in control of my sexual feelings
- Blame—my partner is impulsive, undisciplined, immature
- Distortion 1—anything erotic is threatening (vs. human or arousing)
- Distortion 2—anybody who is sexual is out of control, immoral, base
- Distortion 3—any sexual overture or initiation is exploitive or self-serving (vs. loving or intimate)
- Distortion 4—any sexual desire on my partner's part must be balanced by a greater reserve on my part
- Distortion 5—any sexual issue is immediately suspect

sexual feelings. In this state, anxiety is reduced or eliminated, and compulsive deprivation of any sort is fundamentally about anxiety reduction. But when the anxiety is about sexual terror, the equation is simple. No sex equals no terror. And a powerful sense of well-being accompanies the attainment of an anxiety-free state. The problem is, it does not last.

Inevitably, the transitory well-being is replaced by deep, penetrating despair. A lonely emptiness at the core of the whole process finally asserts itself. "What is wrong with me? Why can't sex and relationships be as easy for me as it seems they are for other people?" At this point, the anorexic senses something is essentially flawed in the equation, and denial gives way to hopelessness and self-hatred. And the anxiety returns.

The "cure" for all of this, of course, is to return to the obsession. Obsessional life blocks the feelings. Focusing on the perceived external threat again becomes an escape from the fearful conclusions of the anorexic's interior world. The distancing strategies are employed again, anxiety levels fall, and the cycle renews itself. Figure 2.2 presents the anorexia cycle.

Figure 2.2

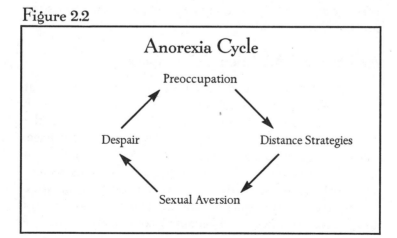

The anorexia cycle requires an extraordinary amount of energy. Anorexics become increasingly unavailable and defensive. Ultimately they treat partners and family members badly, often in ways that they never intended. The control, anger, fear, and impaired thinking take their toll. Business relationships and friendships can also become skewed. They do not survive the anorexic's fear and distortions, and they also become sexualized. There was no sexual content, but the anorexic thought so. And so business decisions and friendship decisions are based on a whole set of rationales that friends and associates have not a clue about. Partners leave as did Shannon's husband of ten years. So do the friends and colleagues. The life of the anorexic becomes unmanageable. It is a trail of broken relationships all of which confirm in the most profound of ways that those original core beliefs were true.

The aversion cycle becomes part of a self-perpetuating system: The core beliefs result in delusional thinking; the impaired thinking supports the aversion cycle; the aversion cycle creates unmanageability; the unmanageability confirms the core beliefs. The sexually anorexic system becomes complete. It feeds on itself, destroying the energy and vitality of the person caught in its power. Figure 2.3 depicts how the system functions.

Anorexia and Addiction: A Comparison

Both sexual anorexics and sex addicts feel powerless. In that sense, the involuntary feelings of aversion in the anorexic are not different from the unwanted feelings of arousal in the addict. They both end up in despair and with great life damage. They both feature delusional thinking that keeps them stuck in what they are doing. They both require maintaining secrets. They are both obsessed with sex. Are we talking about the same illness here? In many ways we are. Chapter 1 described how a compulsive overeater could become a compulsive dieter. The

Figure 2.3

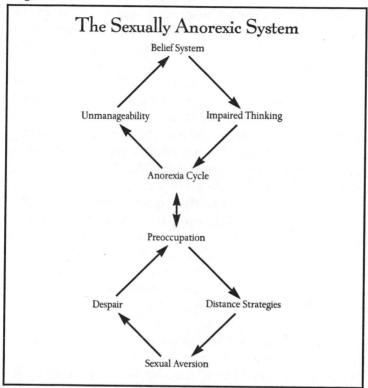

The Sexually Anorexic System

Belief System

Unmanageability · Impaired Thinking

Anorexia Cycle

Preoccupation

Despair · Distance Strategies

Sexual Aversion

same dynamic can occur with sex. This book originated in part from watching recovering sex addicts switch into being compulsively nonsexual. This was not recovery. Sex was still the enemy. There is an interchangeability about the sexual disorders, which Shannon's story illustrates.

After Shannon's first husband left, she fell into a deep depression. She then started an affair with a married man at work. Soon she was cruising bars and having one-night stands. Shannon said, "Within three months I was out of control. I was stunned at how fast it went. From not being able to stand the thought of sex, I went to being obsessed with having it. Affairs and encounters—that's how I spent the next six years." Finally one very tangled affair led to a vicious beating and Shannon was hospitalized. A hospital chaplain finally got Shannon to look at her life, and a week later she sought treatment for her sex addiction. The beating was the wake-up call.

Sex addicts have a very similar behavioral system to that of the sexual anorexics. They have identical core beliefs about being unlovable. The sex addict, however, believes that sex is the most important need—and it can be terrifying or not. This is acceptable because the sex addict's impaired thinking justifies out-of-control sexual behavior. The addict, then, exhibits a cycle similar to the aversion cycle. The addict's obsession with sex leads to rituals that enhance the obsession. The rituals support the sexually compulsive behavior. The addict then feels despair. To cure the despair, the addict returns to the obsession as a way to escape the pain. The content of the system is different—it is the extreme opposite of what the anorexic does—but it has the same components, the same circularity, and the same core assumptions. And often it happens to the same people. Figure 2.4 compares the two systems.

Sexual anorexia must be defined within the context of its companion extreme, just as anorexia nervosa can only be fully understood in terms of its relationship to bulimia or compulsive overeating. The sexual disorders in this sense can be described on a continuum of extremes from the tight, constrained control of the sexual anorexic to the out-of-control behaviors of the sex addict. In between is the area of binge and purge of the sexual bulimic who goes from one extreme to the other. All three conditions draw on the same processes and energy. Not to see this limits our understanding. Thus sex addiction professionals may see addicts go into "recovery" who really have just substituted an anorexic phase of the illness. It is interesting to note that anorexics perceive themselves as very different from the addicts even though, as we have seen, the two dysfunctions draw on the same beliefs and feelings. In fact,

Figure 2.4

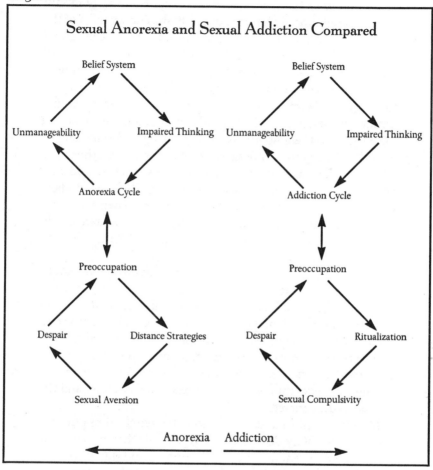

Sexual Anorexia and Sexual Addiction Compared

the anorexics may feel superior to the addicts despite the fact that, as in Shannon's case, their diagnosis could easily change to sex addiction given a different set of circumstances.

None of this is new. History is replete with many examples of all variations of the extremes of our continuum. For example, in the early centuries of the Christian church, both men and women sought lives of deprivation out of religious conviction in order to become more holy. These early monks and nuns renounced all forms of the flesh. The writings of the early desert fathers (the monks and priests of first and second century Christianity) are filled with struggles with sexual desire. Older monks admonished younger monks not only to not think of women but also to not even gaze upon their fellow monks. Examples of success were presented to young ascetics in the form of older monks who had finally achieved mastery over their bodies as evidenced by a certain length period of time with no nocturnal ejaculation. To further their efforts to dominate their sexual impulses, they would also deny themselves sleep, comfort, and food. Thus the eradication of sexual desire was embedded in profound deprivation of all kinds. The irony is that these people were motivated largely by feelings of spiritual inadequacy and unworthiness—much like our contemporary anorexics.[2]

The result was, not surprisingly, torturous obsession—and a fair amount of sexual acting out. Monks commonly sexually abused women and boys sent for spiritual care (bingeing). In fact, an unmarried pregnant woman who did not want to name the father could falsely accuse a monk of paternity—and be believed. Again, there are contemporary parallels. The important things to note, of course, are the commonalties of feelings of unworthiness, the extremes of deprivation, and the fear of sexual contact.

It is important to understand how the switch from purge to binge occurs. Why do some people stay on the anorexic side and others on the addiction side? To understand this, it is essential to look at sexual life in the extremes of the continuum, which is our next chapter.

SEX AS EXTREME

For while there are blatantly acted-out forms of anorexia, there are also quiet, subtle forms of it. Some anorectics may be in no other way addicted. However, beneath the surface, anorexia is a busy addiction: it consists of not doing something, and not doing something, and not doing something. Not trusting. Not committing. Not surrendering.

—Sex and Love Addicts Anonymous[1]

MOST OF US SOONER OR LATER try a diet. We are good for a time and actually start to make progress on our weight loss. And then something happens. A holiday comes up. A stressful series of events. An evening out with friends. Whatever it is, we "fall off the wagon" to use an alcoholism metaphor. Once we start, we may even binge for a while and undo some of our hard-won gains. We may fall into the habit of yo-yo dieting. We diet, lose weight, and put it back on again, maybe even adding some additional pounds. Then we go back on the diet. This is why diets do not work. We do better with informed food choices and exercise. But the process of dieting and bingeing is familiar to most of us.

Therapists have long described the pathological extremes of the binge-purge phenomenon. Perhaps one of the best books on family functioning to come out of the 1980s is entitled *Facing Shame* by family therapists Merle Fossum and Marilyn Mason. The authors describe the binge-purge process as a "shame cycle." Families set high, even unreachable expectations. Kids growing up in such families try to live up to these standards, fail, and try again. They may achieve the family's goals for a while, but inevitably there is failure. When that happens, the children conclude that they are flawed human beings who are unlovable.[2]

Healthy families teach children to feel good about themselves so they can become independent or autonomous. When approval is unreachable, children become ashamed. The famous psychologist Erik Erikson identified this result as "shame versus autonomy." To be locked in shame makes a person vulnerable to all sorts of dependencies. In rigid or disengaged families, this vulnerability often results in the development of the core beliefs discussed in the last chapter. People who grow up in such families experience a loss of self in their unending effort to meet the unreachable standards.[3]

Fossum and Mason describe the unreachable standards as the control side of the shame cycle. Control behaviors include

- compulsive saving
- food anorexia (nervosa)
- sexual anorexia
- compulsive hoarding
- compulsive cleaning
- obligatory exercise
- some phobic responses

Not able to live up to such deprivation extremes, however, people need to act out or get "release" with out-of-control behaviors including

- compulsive violence
- alcoholism
- drug addiction

- sex addiction
- compulsive overeating
- compulsive spending or debting
- workaholism
- compulsive gambling

The release behaviors, however, create great shame. Momentary relief may be found in the acting-out behaviors, but at the price of violating the unreachable standards. So they return to the "control mode," or what therapists often call "acting in." And the cycle starts again. (See figure 3.1)

Figure 3.1

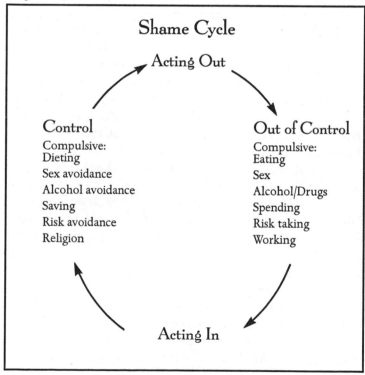

Shame Cycle

Acting Out

Control
Compulsive:
Dieting
Sex avoidance
Alcohol avoidance
Saving
Risk avoidance
Religion

Out of Control
Compulsive:
Eating
Sex
Alcohol/Drugs
Spending
Risk taking
Working

Acting In

When the cycle completes itself over a brief period, we see the binge-purge, or bulimic, phase of the problem. But in many cases the cycle is protracted over time and is therefore less noticeable. A person can also become locked in to the deprivation point or the out-of-control addiction point in the cycle.

Let's use financial behaviors to illustrate the shame cycle. Some people become compulsive spenders whose out-of-control spending is a way to escape their personal pain. The obsession, the purchase, and the initial use are exciting, distracting, and numbing. But soon those feelings begin to fade. A way to avoid despair and shame is to purchase more. The deprivation form of this cycle—the other extreme—is compulsive saving and hoarding. Self-worth is then contingent on how much money is accumulated. No need or comfort is worth the anxiety of not having money.

The binge-purge form of spending disorders combines both extremes. An example would be the professional woman who is caught in this cycle. As a professional, she needs an acceptable wardrobe in which to work. She goes to the department store and buys clothes, usually more than she needs. When she gets home, she starts to regret her buying decisions and feels that she can make do with what she has. She then returns all the merchandise. In fact, she usually has several of these cycles going simultaneously. Instead of having the wardrobe she needs, she has a life of constant turmoil about it.

I met a former patient recently who told me how significant family week had been for him and his family members. Family week is a stage in the treatment process of addictive/compulsive disorders when a patient's entire family comes to stay at the treatment center in order to learn about the family-wide scope of the addiction disease. One of the issues that had been highlighted for them was their financial extremes. The whole family had suffered because of the father's hoarding and saving behaviors. He did not trust banks and would literally count his money each night. And the family would go without. My patient was his son, a sex addict who also had a compulsive spending problem. In fact, his sex addiction was somewhat fused with his compulsive spending in the form of extensive prostitution use. Family week had been a revelation for everyone in the family. For the first time there was frank discussion of money issues. Even so, after family week was over, when the son approached his father about getting together for a cup of coffee, the father said, "I would like to get together with you, but do we have to spend money on coffee?"

The Deprivations

Deprivation draws on two convictions: (1) The deprived person does not believe that he or she is worthy or deserving of pleasure or comfort; and (2) the deprived person feels less anxious and more safe in a deprived state. It is not surprising then that those who suffer compulsive deprivation will seek a number of areas in which to be deprived. Alayne Yates, for example, in her book *Compulsive Exercise and the Eating Disorders* provides extraordinary detail about how excessive dieting and activity disorders can go together. As a physician, she documents how bodybuilders, gymnasts, obligatory (compulsive) runners, and other athletes will combine food anorexia and bulimia with extreme deprivation in the pursuit of the perfect body.[4]

Pioneer sex therapist and physician Domeena Renshaw studied the sexual dysfunction in food anorexics and food bulimics. She found a wide variety of sexual dysfunction including physical issues (such as ceasing of menses and vaginismus) as well as aversive sexual desire.[5] Other researchers found similar kinds of associations including bulimics who would vomit around sexual contact as well as self-cutting and self-mutilation.[6]

Another form of deprivation is compulsive isolation. Sex and Love Addicts Anonymous (SLAA) underlines that along with the sexual deprivation of the sexual anorexic often goes emotional and social deprivation. All forms of human contact can become constricted. Signs of intimacy deprivation noted by SLAA members include

- long periods of no social activities
- feelings of helplessness at being alone
- staying aloof in social groups
- fear of being noticed or recognized
- distant relationships with co-workers
- panic if someone initiates a closer relationship
- discomfort when offered friendship or affection
- dread of being attracted to someone
- attraction only to unavailable or unresponsive persons
- difficulty in playing and having fun with others
- fear of letting people know they matter
- feelings of inadequacy about all relationships
- overwhelmed at the prospect of being honest with others
- fear or resentment toward those who are socially active
- feeling damaged in one's ability to have relationships
- spending time only with family

Such isolation is the logical conclusion of the core beliefs (discussed in the last chapter) when we believe in control. The shame cycle becomes arrested in an existential position based on fear: Do not do or accept anything that would create vulnerability. No chances for mistakes. No chances to be hurt again. No vulnerability. A life stance based on safety—and the denial of human needs.

Mix and Match

Some people, however, mix and match. They will balance deprivation with some excess. And they will do it with the same level of obsession and compulsion. Consider the following examples.

Joan, a thirty-seven-year old single woman, has a problem with compulsive overeating. When she is significantly overweight, she is compulsively nonsexual. Her weight symbolizes her desire to be unattractive. When she loses weight, she starts to act out sexually. Soon she is out of control in one-night stands and affairs. At the height of her sexual acting out she fits all the criteria for food aversion. Joan's weight—either plus or minus one hundred pounds—serves as an index to where she is sexually.

Fran, a forty-five-year-old mother of two, presents a different scenario. She has had four marriages. When married, she would put on about sixty pounds and becomes sexually anorexic. Between marriages she would lose the weight, become a food anorexic, and switch to being sexually addictive. Like Joan, Fran's thinness corresponds to sexual loss of control. The difference is that for Fran, the anorexia phase was contingent on an intimate, married relationship. What finally stopped Fran was the severe sexual violence she suffered at the hands of her last husband. It served a brutal wake-up call; she began to see the pattern of her behavior, and she sought help.

Dale, a fifty-three-year-old attorney, has achieved full partnership in his firm. In fact, his life parallel's the work life described in John Grisham's novels: long torturous hours to generate billable time to gain partnership status. Ninety-hour work weeks are not uncommon even though he is now a partner. To balance his workaholism, Dale has a significant problem with binge spending and advanced alcoholism.

John, in his early fifties, worked ninety-five hours a week as a minister. Attending to the congregation sapped all his strength so that little energy was left for his wife and four kids. He constantly sacrificed his time and efforts for those outside his family, something he felt called to do on the basis of his religious values. The problem was that those sacrifices led him to feel sexually entitled, that he deserved certain sexual rewards. John ended up losing his ministry because of severe sexual misconduct.

These people live in the extremes of the shame cycle. And

the extremes are interactive. Because of their training and background, professional therapists often will focus on a specific presenting problem. Joan told her therapist that her problem was eating. She used to have a problem with "promiscuity," she said, but had not had sex in years. By focusing on the eating disorder, the therapist would have missed the connection with sex. As the eating disorder was treated, however, Joan would have started to lose weight, and then started to act out sexually. The almost certain result is that she would have been filled with shame and dropped out of therapy—and the cycle would have begun again. The bottom line is this: Wherever we demonstrate any excessive behavior, we probably have some balancing behavior that is equally out of control in another direction. Where there is addiction, most likely there will be some kind of deprivation. Where there is deprivation, binge and addictive behavior are present somewhere.

Sometimes we have to look in the family to find the mix and match. Many times I have seen the spouses of sex addicts become increasingly sexually aversive as the addicts progressively became more and more out of control. The more out of control the addict gets, the more shut down the spouse becomes. Similarly, alcoholism researchers in the late 1950s found a group of children of alcoholics who became devoted teetotalers. They were so appalled by what they had seen alcohol do to their parents, they swore they would never use. They became so committed to the idea of abstinence from alcohol that they even found other teetotalers to marry. Many of these people, however, had children who became alcoholics and drug addicts in the early 1970s.

Thus the rhythms of shame and excessive behavior work themselves through a person individually, and also interactively through the family, sometimes over generations. Sex therapists and addiction specialists now know that sexual anorexia seldom appears alone, without associated diagnoses. When the history of the family emerges, it usually forms a complex weave of excesses and deprivations of several types. Addictions and compulsions will revolve in some sort of balance across many generations.

When we conduct family week in a treatment setting, we're often faced with family members reluctant to be present. They are often afraid of family secrets coming out, of the family system being threatened. One of the first things we do is a thorough genogram, or family history, on the board. All family members pool their knowledge to complete it. The result is invariably a profound picture of how the family has been affected by excess and deprivation over many generations. And that every member of the family has been affected. With this realization, family members can often accept the family nature of the disease and commit more fully to family week.

Many therapists are convinced that the shame cycle works at a cultural and social level as well. One of the leaders of trauma medicine research, Sandra L. Bloom, has argued persuasively that people as a community, an ethnic group, or a nation will respond to trauma with excessive or deprivation behaviors in much the same pattern that individual survivors do.[7] So, for example, the bubonic plague traumatized Western Europe. Soon afterward large groups of "flagellants" coursed through European cities, starving and whipping themselves. Similarly, those familiar with financial disorders point to the trauma of the Depression which created a generation of hoarders and compulsive savers followed by a generation of baby boomers who indulged in binge spending.

The Sexual Extremes

Understanding the concept of living in the extremes in general helps immensely when focusing specifically on the sexual extremes. Certain types of extreme sexuality emerge. They are not the only configurations, but they do represent the most common patterns.

Type 1: The Anorexic

In this type, the aversion is complete. Consider the story of Harold. He was the son of a very bright but very shy and retiring inventor. Harold's mother, on the other hand, was loud and boisterous. She was also an alcoholic and a sex addict. She had a number of extramarital affairs and actually had intercourse with Harold when Harold was thirteen. In despair over a career going nowhere and an image of himself as an ineffectual cuckold, Harold's father committed suicide when Harold was ten years old. As an adult, Harold himself was extremely cautious in getting to know people. He went to therapy and became sexually involved with his psychiatrist. They ended up married for two years before breaking up. Harold spent much of his time alone. After his divorce, he did not have sex or date for thirteen years. He did not trust women and felt extremely inadequate as a man. The thought of sex was disgusting to him. He had some experience with masturbation but was deeply troubled by it.

Harold's history contains "classic" components of the sexual anorexic: sexual trauma combined with excessive and deprivation behavior modeled by his parents. He remembered his feelings of anguish as he watched his mother flirt with men at social occasions. When Harold began to acknowledge his anger and understand that he had deserved to be cared for and nurtured as a child, and not betrayed, he began to change. Part of his own deprivation, he came to realize, resulted from a fierce, unconscious loyalty to his father. Becoming sexually involved with his psychiatrist only repeated the profound betrayal in his childhood by his mother. The psychiatrist was yet another caregiver woman who used him. After that experience, Harold had sexually and emotionally shut down in order to avoid further vulnerability. The initial step for him on a journey to sexual healing was finally admitting he had a problem and seeking help.

Sex as Extreme

Type 2: Binge and Purge

As we have seen, there are many forms of binge and purge. However, they all share being sexually out of control at some times and rigidly in control at others. These phases can be sequential as in Fran's case, discussed earlier, in which her binge-purge cycle depended on being married or not married. However, they can be simultaneous as well. An example is the clergyman described in chapter 1 who preached ardently against pornography but who at the same time produced pornography. In his public life he was aversive, and privately he was out of control.

One of the most common forms of simultaneous phases is where an addict is acting out dramatically outside of a committed relationship but within that relationship can only act in—can, in other words, only be compulsively non-sexual. Mick serves as an example. A psychotherapist, Mick had a serious problem with compulsive masturbation. He was masturbating six to eight times a day. He could last about two hours before he had to find a rest room, lock his office door, or go to his car in order to masturbate. He had at times caused significant damage to his genitals because of the aggressiveness with which he pursued this compulsion.

Mick was married to a lovely woman for whom he genuinely cared. She also loved him and felt deep pain because of his lack of sexual responsiveness. Mick told himself that it was because he was so depleted from his "problem," which was in part true. In therapy, however, Mick finally understood that the deeper issue was that he possessed the essential terror of the anorexic, that of combining sexuality and intimacy. Both his mother and grandmother fit the profile of the emotional incest syndrome—provocative, intrusive, overwhelming, and exploitive. Their narcissistic use of him to make their lives complete caused a deep sense of the need for self-protection in Mick. To live in the fantasy world of compulsive masturbation was safe in its unreality. To love his wife, but not be sexual with her, could also be made safe. The idea of combining the two, however, filled Mick with abject fear.

The family histories of sexual anorexics and addicts may vary, and the forms of acting out might change. What is common for many, however, is acting out—or acting in—sexually while avoiding sexual intimacy. This has been seen in sex addicts in general.[8] It has also been described as common in the various paraphilias, including voyeurism, exhibitionism, and fetishism.[9] And it has been documented repeatedly in sex offenders.[10] They all have in common a tremendous fear of sex and intimacy. They are also often tormented by self-hatred because they feel so flawed.

Type 3: The Addictive Switch

In alcoholism, a phenomenon exists called the "dry drunk." For any number of reasons, the alcoholic switches to not drinking. He or she may, in fact, become a proselytizer against alcohol. But the essential features that supported out-of-control drinking remain: rigid judgmentalism, unforgiving shame, and profound feelings of unworthiness. Recovering people have long recognized that alcoholism persists even in people who no longer drink. An alcoholic's suffering can bring about, however, a deep transformation of the self. That is what recovery is. Without recovery, the immediate possibility of switching back always lurks close by.

The same pattern occurs with sex. Some people spend a portion of their lives acting out sexually. Then they switch and become anorexics. The same core beliefs remain intact, however, and they may even preach against sexual excess. Many of the early leaders of the Christian church appear to be operating in that mode. St. Augustine, for example, in his *Confessions* describes a period of sexual acting out in his life and then argues for a life of temperance and abstinence. In addition to reflecting the culture in which he lived and wrote, Augustine's story is an example of the addictive switch.

The addictive-switch type of sexual anorexic/addict mainly comprises sex addicts who enter recovery, but who remain in the dry drunk, or anorexic, mode. There is no forgiveness of self or others in this "recovery." There does remain, however, an unrelenting obsession with and fear of their sexuality, which is reinforced by the tremendous damage caused by their previous, excessive sexual behavior. It is almost as if they have been so traumatized by what they have done that sex in any guise becomes the abuser, the enemy.

I once attended a convention of sex addicts in which a man got up and in tears told everyone his story. He had been free from sexually acting out for four years. In great pain and anguish he confessed that he now had to start over because he had a wet dream. Fortunately, he was surrounded by loving people who helped him to see that he was being extremely hard on himself. The man still had no compassion for his journey nor had he developed a love for himself as a sexual being.

Type 4: The Anorexic Partner

Sometimes people become sexually anorexic because of a traumatizing relationship. Michelle learned that her husband, Fred, was having affairs when one of the seven women he was simultaneously involved with wrote her a letter telling her of what had been happening. At one level she was not surprised. Her husband was so demanding of her sexually that some nights she would actually sneak out and sleep in the family's car. It was the one place she could go, lock the doors, and feel safe. When they did have sex, he was so rough and assaultive that her body would be bruised, and her breasts and genitals would be sore. She felt trapped because with children she did not have the financial means to leave. She found sex repulsive. She felt completely isolated and too ashamed to tell anyone.

Finally, a neighbor out for an early morning walk found her asleep in the car. This lovely, older woman was afraid that something had happened to Michelle such as carbon monoxide poisoning so she woke Michelle up. Somehow her neighbor's concern opened the door for Michelle. Sitting on the sidewalk next to the car she sobbed in the woman's arms. The neighbor bundled Michelle up and took her to her pastor. Soon she was in a shelter for battered women with her children. It took a long time for Michelle to get comfortable with her sexuality. The alert pastor got her into therapy and the husband into treatment for sex addiction. Sadly, the marriage did not survive, which was painful for the children. But Michelle did get into recovery for herself. She later described that morning sitting by the car sharing tears with her neighbor as the waking from the nightmare.

There is no doubt that some partnerships are traumatic. Clearly, some people become anorexic in response to their partner's excessive behavior.

Type 5: Simultaneous Anorexia

Sometimes both partners will be sexually anorexic. The scenario goes like this: Two people grow up very wounded emotionally and sexually. They are attracted to each other and like the companionship. They also like the fact that the other has no desire for sex. So part of their original covenant together is not to be sexual—or at least very sexual. As time goes by, however, they each become aware of some emptiness in their lives.

Larry and Chris have a story like that. Chris came from a rigid Catholic family with no-talk rules about sex. At age sixteen, while babysitting, she found some pornography and was aroused by it. She masturbated using the pornography but then was filled with shame. She was tortured by obsessive images of God cutting her finger off because of the masturbation. She and Larry had two boys, and she saw this as God's punishment as well since she did not want to deal with boys and their sexuality. She had wanted girls instead.

Larry's background was similar. When he was five, he was horribly abused sexually by a neighbor. His father and grandfather were both alcoholics and his mother was a raging codependent. His mother walked in on him once while he was masturbating, which resulted in an angry scene. For years she tried to catch him masturbating again. Even in high school she would rip the shower curtain back to see if he was playing with himself in the shower. She never caught him again, but she always made some shaming comment nonetheless.

In Chris and Larry's marriage, sex went from infrequent to nonexistent. It was a sexual standoff. Neither initiated. Through a group for adult children of alcoholics Larry learned about Recovering Couples Anonymous (RCA). With the help of a therapist and supportive RCA couples, Larry and Chris started to give themselves permission for sexual feelings. They actually began to have romantic feelings for each other. They both agreed that two years of being with supportive couples were like a miracle in reclaiming their sexual lives separately and together.

The aphorism of "opposites attract" is often true. But many therapists have also seen how both partners will often come from the same type of family system. There is an attraction to the safety of the familiar. There is also a bond that can exist in shared terror—even if it is unspoken.

Type 6: Simultaneous Binge and Purge

The pattern of sexual bingeing outside of the relationship while being sexually aversive in the relationship can be true for both partners. Tim and Karen were like that. Tim was acting out in xxx-rated video stores and with prostitutes. It was dangerous sex because it was often unprotected sex and often in high-risk situations. He virtually ignored Karen sexually. Karen was quite righteous about the risks Tim took and his emotional and sexual absence in the relationship.

In family week, however, it became clear that Karen was very similar. She had entered the sexual intrigue of the Internet and loved it. She would find herself still into it at five in the morning wondering where the night had gone. She spent long periods in chat rooms and bulletin boards having sexually explicit conversations. From there, she graduated to giving her phone number to men she met in cyberspace. Phone sex gave way to personal meetings at beaches and motels. When pressed, she had to admit there was very little difference between what she was doing sexually and what Tim was doing. Both were high-risk situations. She further had to admit that in Tim's presence her sexual desire had long been gone. The truth was that it was easier to play the abandoned lover than to admit that she had left the relationship too.

The problem was that Tim and Karen genuinely cared for one another. And they had two small children to whom they were devoted. Recovery was painful at times, agonizing for both, but they also found an RCA group, and within six months they found themselves recommitted to working on the relationship. One year later they were starting to trust the changes they were making.

Sexual Anorexia, Addiction, and Codependency

We must now separate the concepts of sexual anorexia, sexual addiction, and co-sex addiction, or codependency. Many thousands of scholarly articles exist documenting addiction as a family illness. In the case of alcoholism or compulsive gambling, spouses and family members become obsessed with the addict's loss of control. They obsess about the addict's behavior, torture themselves with feelings of responsibility for what is happening, and attempt to control the addict—all of which simply makes the problem worse. Codependents lose touch with their own needs and feelings, thus becoming alienated from themselves.

Excellent books exist describing codependency and sex addiction. Jennifer Schneider, for example, in her book *Back from Betrayal* describes how betrayal affects the sexuality of the codependent partner.[11] Like other codependents, co-sex addicts are obsessed with the addict's behavior. The difference is that compared with other codependents, the co-sex addict is often more intense. If our partner chooses a bottle or a slot machine rather than us, there will be hurt and anguish. But if our partner chooses other women or men rather than us, the hurt and anguish are amplified by profound feelings of sexual rejection and abandonment.

Sexual dependency shares the same kinds of internal mechanisms that create problems for the addict and the anorexic. Codependents have the same core beliefs about being unworthy and unlovable. They have elaborate rationalizations for their various efforts to change the addict. They are often in denial about themselves as well as the addict. Their codependent behavior such as lying to cover up what the addict has done creates tremendous unmanageability. The lives of codependents are filled with obsession and preoccupation as well. The difference is how codependents view sex. They have a core belief that sex is the most important sign of love. In *Out of the Shadows,* I describe this belief as the driving force behind the obsession with the addict. The codependent concludes, "If my partner is sexual with someone else and not me, I am for sure not lovable." Terror and anxiety about abandonment rule the co-sex addict's life.

Sexual anorexia can also be central to codependent obsession. There can be co-anorexia. If the partner drags the anorexic who is in denial to see a therapist in order to change the anorexic into sexual responsiveness, the preoccupation is no different than when the co-addict drags the addict into treatment. Co-anorexics may conclude that their sexual problems are their fault, that they are not sexy or desirable enough—which are the same conclusions co-addicts reach in order to explain their partners' behavior. Efforts to coerce and control the anorexic into sexual responsiveness are as effective as the co-addict's efforts to control the addict.

Figure 3.2 Core Beliefs for Three Obsessional States of Mind

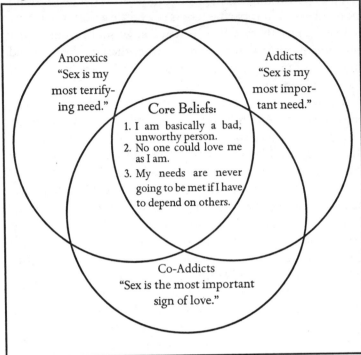

Anorexics
"Sex is my most terrify- ing need."

Addicts
"Sex is my most impor- tant need."

Core Beliefs:

1. I am basically a bad, unworthy person.
2. No one could love me as I am.
3. My needs are never going to be met if I have to depend on others.

Co-Addicts
"Sex is the most important sign of love."

Figure 3.2 graphically illustrates how the three obsessional states draw on the same core beliefs about unworthiness, unlovability, and distrust. The obsession shifts according to which belief has predominance. Thus addiction, anorexia, and codependency are all separate and definable. However, it is common for a co-addict to be anorexic but not always. Some co-addict's sexual desire can remain unaffected or even amplified in the presence of a sex addict. A sex addict can be co-anorexic attempting to push an anorexic partner into sexual responsiveness. Some anorexics are neither codependent nor addictive. A good number of people are all the above.

The recovery lesson here is this: It is very important to see that we are describing variations of a theme. Neither the addiction

nor the anorexic extremes can be defined without understanding the relationship between them. Nor can they be understood without examining the family relationships because the
extremes appear there as well. If we throw in other forms of
deprivation and excess, the resulting mosaic of extreme behavior tells us how pain and anxiety are managed.

The core beliefs remain as the foundation for all the variations of sexual obsession. The differences are really about fear.
Sex addicts are afraid they will miss out on sex that will make
them whole. Anorexics are afraid that if they are sexual, they
will experience how empty and hurting they are. Co-addicts
are afraid of being left alone because of sex. Which obsession
will dominate? That depends on what the individual is most
afraid of.

Trauma and Fear

Since the early 1980s therapists have made extraordinary
progress in understanding posttraumatic stress disorder. Here
is a summary of key discoveries:

1. *Survivors of trauma tend to process information in the extremes.* An alter-
   ation occurs in the biological strata of the brain that causes
   survivors to overreact to stress and threat. They will go to
   one extreme or another to prevent further trauma. On one
   end they may "freeze" somewhat, as an animal does to
   avoid discovery. On the other hand, they may go into
   extreme activity to cope with what is happening. They have
   trouble finding a middle-ground approach.

2. *Trauma is a powerful factor in the genesis of addictions and compulsions.*
   A wealth of data show trauma as a factor in deprivation.
   Trauma specialists describe this as "traumatic abstinence."
   Similarly, addictions serve often as a maladaptive solution
   to the trauma. Addiction can take the form of high arousal
   or pleasure as an antidote to pain, or an effort to numb

anxiety, or as escape from reality. Sometimes survivors will repeat the trauma in some form to achieve the same neurochemical responses they had during the original events. When this occurs, that addiction is to the trauma, what clinicians call "repetition compulsion."

3. *Trauma does not have to be a specific event.* Living in a rigid or disengaged family can be traumatic for a child. Being around an alcoholic or addict of any type can be traumatic. Neglect can have a profound impact. Anything that induces extreme shame can be traumatic.

4. *Fear can have a profound impact on sexual development.* Terror can totally shut down sexual development right at the point the terror was experienced. Extreme fear can also serve as an escalator to sex, especially if the survivor experienced pleasure and fear at the same time. A mental template is formed in which the adult seeks dangerous sex. For example, a woman abused physically and sexually as a child might be able to be orgasmic only if a man is hurting her. Some people have had both experiences, the shut-down experience and the high-risk arousal.

Trauma and addiction specialists are finding common ground regarding the nature of these problems. Understanding the role of fear in the sexual extremes helps us to understand what people have to go through to reclaim their sexuality. As the stories in this chapter have shown, the mosaic of extremes is really about fear. To heal will require an environment of safety and nurturing. The core beliefs must be undermined. A new relationship with self has to emerge. And impaired thinking about sex will have to be set aside to reduce false or mythic fears. This is a process almost like growing up all over again. And, eventually, healing will require facing the real risk: What can happen when we combine genuine intimacy and our sexual vulnerability.

SEX AS HEALING

My illusive tools for survival, gifts from some primeval ances-tor, passed in secret along the chain of my forebears. In the end, mine is a navigator's sense of place and the strength again to hoist the sails, the will again to catch the winds; and even when the land and all that I ever loved are lost to me, and the stars are shrouded, and I am sore with losses, and afraid—even then, the miracles all around leap to celebrate themselves, and I will celebrate them too. And even then, I'll trust that a new shore will rise to meet me, and there in that new place, I will find new things to care about.

—Mia Farrow, *What Falls Away*

WHEN I MET DEEDEE, the first thing she told me was, "I was both a mother and a wife by the time I was eleven." I asked her how this could be and the story unfolded. Deedee's mother went to work when Deedee was eleven and Deedee took over the care of her younger brother who was five. She also took over many of the household chores. Her mother's absence was a symbol of something deeper than financial stress. Her mother was also having a series of affairs. Dad and Mom were sleeping in separate bedrooms. Deedee became a companion to her father. She was his confidant. He even took her dancing at the American

Legion club. At the time, she thought it was great. Much later, with years of pain and the accumulated perspective of extensive therapy, she saw it for what it was. She had become the surrogate wife. She told me sadly, "I have very little memory of being a child. I have this photograph of me as a kid standing there with a little Christmas tree. I have no memory of it."

Deedee's dad was never overtly sexual with her. But her mom sensed the emotional bond and was jealous. Deedee's parents would fight about how to discipline her. If Dad was not severe enough, Mom would add to the consequences. And then her parents would fight more about it. They divorced when Deedee was fifteen. A few years later her mom, in a night of sorrowful drinking, told Deedee about all her affairs and extramarital sex. Retrospectively, Deedee concluded her mom was terribly out of control. After the divorce, however, Deedee's mom switched to the anorexic side. She never again went out with a man.

After the divorce, Deedee ran away from her dad's house. The good news is that she found refuge with her boyfriend's parents. To this day, she is grateful for their kindness. The bad news is that the boyfriend was sexually abusive to her. He would create elaborate sexual scenarios that often were painful. He would buy boots for her and have her walk on him. Years later, Deedee's therapist observed that it was really Deedee who was being walked on. Deedee went home to her dad and brother, but now she knew about drugs. Deedee found other abusive men and experienced date rape a number of times. Since she was always high, she did not think it mattered.

Then Sandy came into her life. He was a handsome musician in a band on the verge of making it. Like a groupie, Deedee manipulated her way into meeting him. There was an instant chemistry fueled by sex and drugs. They spent their first week together high and in bed. Then they married and sex disappeared. After their two children were born, they went almost nine years having intercourse two to three times a year. The desire was gone.

Part of the problem was Sandy. He described his family as an "emotional refrigerator." No touching. No talk about sex. No feelings. His outlet became music, drugs, and sex in that order. As long as he was high, he could do anything—and did. Groupies, voyeurism, and compulsive masturbation. He remembers with addictive pride being stoned at the Boston Marathon watching the women runners go by and playing "pocket pool"—masturbating over and over again.

Deedee did not know about Sandy's sexual acting out until much later. She did know that something was wrong. Drugs were ruining their life together. When her older daughter was four and her second daughter was six months old, Deedee realized that for their sake she and Sandy had to change. She arranged for an intervention on Sandy and voluntarily went to treatment herself. Recovery from drugs changed their lives. Things got much better. They worked on their individual recoveries. But sex remained taboo. Without drugs, they were resigned to being companions.

Deedee saw a *Donahue* show on sex addiction. Having just returned to therapy, she shared her reactions with her new therapist. Her therapist helped her to see how the rhythms of deprivation and excess were part of Sandy and Deedee's married life. Deedee and Sandy both agreed that the real changes occurred for them when they started looking at their sexual issues. They realized that they had entered what her therapist called an "anorexic covenant." The basic components of that contract were (1) no sexual demands of one another; (2) no risk or instability after the chaos of the past; and (3) an accommodation with general unhappiness. Her therapist categorized the last part as a "pact for misery."

Doing a "first step" in regard to her sexual anorexia transformed Deedee. From the perspective of Twelve Step programs, the First Step is an inventory of feelings of powerlessness and

unmanageability. Deedee shared in a women's group how helpless she was over her feelings of sexual aversion and how her
feelings had made her life extremely hard. She realized how any
gesture of affection or touch from Sandy would put her
instantly on guard for any sexual agenda he might have.
Beginning with her father, she had always worried about what
men wanted. Without drugs, however, she could not stand the
anxiety. And she hated herself for it.

Deedee and Sandy also started going to a Recovering
Couples Anonymous/RCA group. Sandy saw that decision as
having a profound impact on their sexuality. The turning
point was when one of their children had a medical crisis. They
were immediately surrounded by loving RCA couples who
brought food and helped them out. Deedee admitted she had
a terrible time accepting their nurturing. "I was supposed to be
a giver, not a receiver," she sighed. Accepting care was so hard.
If she did accept care in her family, it meant choosing between
her mom and her dad. It was much more comfortable taking
care of everyone else. Remember, Deedee had been both a
mother and wife by the age of eleven.

With the group's help, she realized she was worthy of care.
With her therapist's help, she realized that she could accept
sexual nurturing. In fact, she told me laughingly, "When we
heard you were looking for couples from our RCA group to be
interviewed for a book on healthy sexuality, we all laughed and
joked about who knew what that was. But I thought about it
for a second and realized, I did now know. The last two years
have been unbelievable. I feel so free and trusting." Deedee
had discovered an essential truth: Facing sexual issues can
work wonderful and profound changes in who we are.

The Healing Journey

The healing journey starts with admitting there is a problem.
Remember that denial is core to the impaired thinking
process. Confronting sexual anorexia is hard to do alone or

even with a loving partner. That is why therapists can be so helpful. They are trained to help put things in perspective. There is too much about sexual anorexia—parent issues, residual feelings from past trauma, addiction issues, living in a sex-negative culture—that make it difficult to resolve by oneself.

Finding a therapist can be a challenge. What is needed is a good therapist who has a thorough grounding in addiction issues, sexual medicine, trauma therapy, and family of origin work. Sometimes local treatment facilities and professional associations can make helpful recommendations. Members in a Twelve Step network usually know who the better therapists are. Pastors, too, can make good recommendations. They are often the ones people go to first for help, and they make many referrals. At the beginning of this book is an 800-number to call for recommendations for therapists in almost every city in North America.

This chapter includes an inventory to assist individuals in organizing their thoughts prior to seeing a therapist. It reflects the First Step of Twelve Step programs: "We admitted we were powerless over [sexual aversion]—that our lives had become unmanageable." As such, the inventory might be used in a group setting or in a Twelve Step context. The purpose of the inventory is to increase self-knowledge, which is, along with admitting the existence of a problem, the starting point for the healing journey.

✐ SEXUAL ANOREXIA INVENTORY

SECTION 1: SIGNS OF ANOREXIA AND DEPRIVATION

Please check all the following that are true for you now or have been true for you sometime in your past.

SIGNS OF SEXUAL ANOREXIA:

___ 1.   Dread of sexual pleasure

___ 2.   Persistent fear of sexual contact

___ 3.   Obsessive vigilance about sexual matters

___ 4.   Avoidance of anything connected with sex

___ 5.   Preoccupation with other people being sexual

___ 6.   Distortions about your own body's appearance

___ 7.   Extreme loathing of body functions

___ 8.   Obsessional self-doubt about sexual adequacy

___ 9.   Rigid, judgmental attitudes about sexual behavior

___ 10.   Excessive fear and preoccupation with sexually transmitted diseases

___ 11.   Obsessive concern or worry about the sexual intentions of others

___ 12.   Shame and self-loathing over sexual experiences

___ 13.   Despair about sexual adequacy and functioning

___ 14.   Avoiding intimacy because of sexual fear

___ 15.   Self-destructive behavior to limit, stop, or avoid sex

SIGNS OF EMOTIONAL AND SOCIAL DEPRIVATION

___ 1.   Long periods of no social activities

___ 2.   Feelings of helplessness at being alone

___ 3.   Staying aloof in social groups

___ 4.   Fear of being noticed or recognized

___ 5.   Distant relationships with co-workers

___ 6.   Panic if someone initiates a closer relationship

___ 7.   Discomfort when offered friendship or affection

___ 8.   Dread of being attracted to someone

___ 9.   Attraction to unavailable or unresponsive persons

___10.   Difficulty in playing and having fun with others

___11.   Fear of letting other people know they matter

___12.   Feelings of inadequacy about all relationships

___13.   Overwhelmed at the prospect of being honest with
          others

___14.   Fear or resentment for those who are socially active

___15.   Feeling damaged in your ability to have relationships

COLLATERAL DEPRIVATIONS

___ 1.   Anorexia nervosa (food)

___ 2.   Compulsive saving

___ 3.   Compulsive hoarding

___ 4.   Compulsive cleaning

___ 5.   Obligatory or excessive exercise

___ 6. Phobic responses

___ 7. Perfectionism

___ 8. Obsessive compulsive behavior

___ 9. Workaholism (as depletion and avoidance)

COLLATERAL ADDICTIVE OR BINGE BEHAVIOR

___ 1. Sex addiction

___ 2. Compulsive violence

___ 3. Drug addiction

___ 4. Alcoholism

___ 5. Compulsive overeating

___ 6. Compulsive spending or debting

___ 7. Workaholism (as excitement and involvement)

___ 8. Compulsive gambling

SECTION 2: KEY QUESTIONS

Please answer the following questions as completely as you can. Remember, you do not have to respond perfectly. The goal is to assemble your thoughts in a thorough way. You can answer one question at a time and take breaks in between. Be gentle with yourself as this may be difficult. Write your answers on a separate sheet of paper.

1. Are you codependent? That means, do you spend a great deal of time and energy taking care of others and obsessing about their behavior?

2. Do you have family members who are addicts of some type? Do any of your family members have deprivation behavior? List their names and their behaviors.

3. List examples in your life when you were not sexual when you wanted to be.

4. List examples in your life when you were sexual and had no desire to be so.

5. Describe some of the primary things you might do to avoid sexual contact.

6. Give at least three examples of obsessing about sex and how to avoid it. For example, *I worry constantly that my [husband, wife, partner] is going to touch me, so I'm always alert to not providing an opportunity for it to happen.*

7. Describe some of your greatest losses as a result of your sexual deprivation. What feelings do you have about them now?

8. In what ways have you lied, covered up, or minimized your aversion to sex?

9. In what ways did you try to explain, rationalize, or justify your feelings about sex?

10. In what ways have you denied you have a problem?

11. How have your sexual feelings affected your self-esteem?

12. In what ways have you tried to manipulate others so as not to have to be sexual?

13. What hobbies, interests, or friends have you given up as a result of your obsession with avoiding sexual issues?

SECTION 3:
POWERLESSNESS AND UNMANAGEABILITY

POWERLESSNESS

Powerlessness means being unable to stop feelings of sexual aversion despite the consequences this has for you. On a separate sheet of paper, list as many examples of sexual avoidance as you can. Be as explicit and concrete as possible. Example: *I would deliberately start a fight with my spouse so there was no possibility of our getting amorous.* Start with you earliest examples and conclude with your most recent. By giving as many examples as possible, you will add significantly to your understanding of your own powerlessness. That understanding is essential to recovery.

You do not have to complete this in one sitting. Add to the list as examples occur to you. Get support from others as you work on it.

UNMANAGEABILITY

In addition to being powerless over involuntary aversion to sex, most people describe negative life results, a feeling that their whole lives are chaotic, hectic, and built on false foundations.

On a separate sheet of paper, list as many examples as you can think of that show how your life has become chaotic, damaged, or unmanageable because of your sexual anorexia. Example: *I lied to escape a date with a man I genuinely liked. He found out, was angry, and I never saw him again.* Again be gentle with yourself. Remember to call your therapist or group members as you go through this. You deserve to have support.

CONSEQUENCES

Whenever there is compulsive deprivation, there is a price to pay. We call these consequences. They are not always so obvious with sexual anorexia. Here is a list of consequences other anorexics have reported as part of their experience. Check the ones that fit you.

___ 1. Thoughts or feelings about committing suicide

___ 2. Attempted suicide

___ 3. Homicidal thoughts or feelings

___ 4.   Feelings of hopelessness and despair

___ 5.   Feeling like you have two lives—one public and one secret

___ 6.   Depression, paranoia, or fear of going insane

___ 7.   Loss of touch with reality

___ 8.   Loss of self-esteem

___ 9.   Loss of life goals

___ 10.   Acting against your own values and beliefs

___ 11.   Strong feelings of guilt and shame

___ 12.   Strong feelings of isolation and shame

___ 13.   Strong fears for your future

___ 14.   Emotional exhaustion

___ 15.   Extreme weight loss or gain

___ 16.   Physical problems (ulcers, high blood pressure, etc.)

___ 17.   Physical injury or abuse

___ 18.   Involvement in potentially abusive or dangerous situations

___ 19.   Sleep disturbance

___ 20.   Physical exhaustion

___ 21.   Feelings of spiritual emptiness

___ 22.   Feeling disconnected from yourself and the world

___ 23.   Feeling abandoned by God or your Higher Power

___ 24.   Anger at God or your Higher Power

___ 25. Loss of faith in anything spiritual

___ 26. Risking loss of partner or spouse

___ 27. Loss of partner or spouse

___ 28. Increase in marital or relationship problems

___ 29. Loss of partner's or spouse's respect

___ 30. Problems with children

On a separate sheet of paper, record your reactions and feelings about these consequences. What has been the impact of sexual deprivation on your life?

Finding a Group

Another important part of the healing process is to find a support group. Sexual anorexics are welcome at all Sex and Love Addicts Anonymous (SLAA) meetings. In many cities, SLAA or one of the other sex-addiction fellowships sponsor groups just for anorexics.

Recovering Couples Anonymous (RCA) is also a wonderful forum for working on these issues. Deedee and Sandy found the weekly support of other couples in recovery indispensable. Sandy pointed out that neither he nor Deedee had a model for how a couple should be together. The only requirement to join an RCA group is that one of the partners has had some Twelve Step experience such as Alcoholics Anonymous, Gamblers Anonymous, or Overeaters Anonymous. Any of the codependency programs also qualify, including Al-Anon, S-Anon (partners' group for Sexaholics Anonymous), Co-Sex Addicts Anonymous (partners' group for Sex Addicts Anonymous), or Adult Children of Alcoholics Anonymous. Recovering Couples Anonymous is a receptive and supportive fellowship that is showing people how to make Twelve Step principles work in their lives. If you are in a committed relationship, RCA could make a significant contribution to your sexual healing together. If you are not in a relationship, it can help a great deal when you do start one.

Therapists also have therapy group options for their clients. Combining a self-help group such as SLAA with group therapy optimizes chances for staying in balance. Also, many treatment facilities for inpatient care offer sexual disorder tracks that have been critical for people to get started.

The important thing for sexual anorexics is to start laying the foundation of a supportive community for their journey. They will have to confront issues about who they are, how their family was, and what unresolved trauma and abuse still reside in their unconscious. The goal here is overcoming sexual self-hatred. The remainder of this book is designed to guide the sexual anorexic—and indeed anyone who wishes a healthy sexuality—toward that release. But for this to happen, we will need all the support we can muster.

SEX AS HEALTH

To sum up about sex: We earnestly pray for the right ideal, for guidance in each questionable situation, for sanity, and for the strength to do the right thing.
— The "Big Book" of Alcoholics Anonymous

CHANGE. How does real change happen? Usually it only occurs if the system changes. Understanding how systems work has revolutionized how we look at change. We rely on systems to function as they are supposed to. The solar system. Weather systems. Computer systems. Arterial systems. They are predictable and repetitive. Behavior, too, is part of some system, predictable and repetitive. Sometimes, however, a behavior system does not work for us and then we need to change it. Unless we understand how that system functions, our efforts may only make things worse.

Consider the woman who marries the same type of abusive alcoholic three times. Has she changed? For sure she has changed husbands. Yet her life remains stuck in the same ways. The irony here is that each time she remarried, she was looking to do better. She wanted an upgrade. Yet what happened—as is often the case—was that the next husband was worse than the last. It seemed like the harder she tried the worse her life got.

Therapists call this "first-order change," as in the aphorism, "the more things change the more they remain the same." This woman has not changed the system she is in. But suppose that she goes to a therapist for help and the therapist urges her to join a women's group. The woman has a hard time with this because she distrusts other women. But she learns in the group that other women can be trustworthy. She discovers that many of the things she was seeking from men she could get from women. Companionship. Care. Nurturing. She takes a "time-out" from dating. She starts to understand her family of origin. She learns that she came from an alcoholic family and that the way she is attracted to men guarantees abusive, alcoholic partners. With the help of others, she concludes that she is worthy of better. Her life changes. Her next partner is dramatically different—and for the better.

When the system is fundamentally altered, therapists call this "second-order change." To achieve this type of change, the rules of the system must change. In a computer system, we must change the programming. In a family system, we must change the family rules. In individuals, we must change our beliefs. Most people have problems because they believe in certain solutions. The harder they try the solutions that do not work, the more stuck they become. It is another way to understand insanity. It is insanity to continue doing things that do not work. But it is very systemic. [1]

Anorexia and addiction are first-order phenomena. They are predictable, repetitive, and resistant to change. The harder addicts try to stop, the more out of control they become. The more anorexics try to make sex work for them, the more elusive it becomes. Family members or partners who try to control and change the anorexic or the addict make things worse. Remember, that excess and deprivation are anchored in a cycle of shame. We can switch addictions. We can find different ways to be deprived, but the essential system will remain intact.

Stephen Covey describes the change process in his classic *Seven Habits of Highly Effective People.*[2] He points out that if we focus on a specific behavior, we can achieve modest change. Significant change only occurs if there is a paradigm shift. In other words, second-order change will happen if the programming is altered. The belief system must be dismantled and rebuilt. Any therapy that focuses simply on sex or specific behaviors and does not involve a shift in perception will fail.

Anorexics believe in control and safety. Their core beliefs tell them they can only rely on themselves because of their unworthiness and unlovability. They believe sex is dangerous and high risk so they try to repress it. They want intimacy but fear it is unreachable for them. So they focus on preventing abandonment. They have dysfunctional beliefs about their own sex and the opposite sex. They have been programmed to present an invulnerable face to the external world.

Sex addicts believe they have to have sex, but they, too, must keep it secret because of their fear. Fear for them just makes sex more compelling. They share with anorexics the same false ideas about men, women, and intimacy. They have different externals but the same shadow side. The core beliefs embed them in the same shame and conviction of their fundamental unworthiness. The anorexic and the addict must deal with the core issues in order to experience the deep change of the paradigm shift. Otherwise they will simply switch from one form of the obsession to the other. Or stay stuck.

In Twelve Step fellowships, change starts with the First Step. When anorexics admit that by themselves they are not able to change, that they need help, they make a leap into a new paradigm. The admission of powerlessness undermines the tyranny of the old core beliefs. Anorexics learn that other people care and that they do not have to undergo change alone. Further, they can have support and not have it mean that they are vulnerable to abuse or exploitation.

Some people and even some professionals interpret powerless to mean helpless. They fear that such language gives permission for irresponsibility. On the contrary, the First Step is an admission that the old solutions do not work no matter how hard we try them. A First Step done well is an incredible act of courage. At the same moment, the anorexic allows tremendous vulnerability and takes extraordinary responsibility by following the one route that is still available: asking for help. All painfully learned rules about safety, protection, perfectionism, and control have to be set aside. Experienced therapists call this a "paradoxical intervention." Anorexics do not need to try harder. That is part of their problem. They need to let go and trust. Figure 5.1 illustrates the paradigm shift from the old rules to the new.

Figure 5.1

The Paradigm Shift		
First-Order Changes	P	Second-Order Changes
Anorexics believe:	A	Recovery creates new beliefs:
• That they are unworthy and unloveable	R	
• That they cannot depend on others	A	• That they are precious and loveable
• That they will have to take care of themselves	D	• That others will help them meet their needs
• That relationships make them vulnerable to abuse and exploitation	I G M	• That they can have support
		• That relationships do not have to be abusive or exploitive
• That sex is terrifying	S	• That sex can be safe and loving
• That sex must be controlled and repressed	H	
• That intimacy and sex cannot be combined	I	• That sex is an authentic expression of self
	F	• That sex works best when there is healthy bonding
	T	

Toward a Healthy Sexuality

Central to the paradigm shift for anorexics will be a new understanding of their sexuality. They will learn to see sex as an authentic expression of self that can be safe and loving. They will also confront their biggest fear which is to combine intimacy and sex. They will discover sex actually works best when there is healthy bonding.

In this sense, we see one more parallel with the eating disorders. Compulsive overeaters and food anorexics in recovery do not give up food. They learn how to eat differently. They learn about their emotional relationship to food and how they have misused food. They will choose different kinds of foods. They have a food plan based on what is healthy for them. In fact, our current consciousness about healthy eating in many ways has emerged out of our understanding of eating disorders.

I believe that a sexual consciousness will also emerge from our understanding of sexual disorders. For many years professionals have stumbled around about what goes into a healthy sexuality. Books and articles on healthy relationships are legion. There are tens of thousands of research articles about the nature of sexual problems. There are thousands of articles about sexual physical functioning and how to correct dysfunctions, whether or not they are organic in nature. And there is much available regarding controversies surrounding sex-related topics such as gay rights, feminism, sex education, and contraception. However, there are relatively few professionals who have come forward and said, "This is what healthy sex looks like."

One of those pioneering spirits is family researcher James Maddock. Building on the guidelines evolved under the auspices of the World Health Organization, Maddock constructed a model of healthy sexuality in the family. He identifies five key factors:

- A healthy family finds a balanced interdependence of males and females who are equally respected with shared power and control.
- A healthy family creates a balance through boundaries that define individuality yet permit physical and emotional closeness.
- A healthy family facilitates communication that enhances—but also distinguishes—nurturing, affection, and erotic contact.
- A healthy family helps members develop sexual values, meanings, and attitudes that are shared, and supports individuals if they differ.
- A healthy family defines itself as a unique sexual system that can agree or disagree with community, family of origin, and culture but remain connected to those groups.

Most important, Maddock sees the family as an environment in which healthy sexuality is taught, supported, and nurtured.[3]

Sex therapist Ginger Manley similarly has defined a model of healthy sexuality that builds on gender equality, relational ability, and personal integrity. In writing about sexual health and recovery from sexual addiction, she also underlines the role of meaning and spirituality. She describes the movement away from a "shame-based" sexuality in which sex exists in a continuum "from aversive to immersive—or from acting in to acting out." Since shame is built on disgrace, the new model of sexual health should be built on a sense of grace—put in other words, a sense of empowerment and connection with self and others. Manley sees many of Maddock's components for a healthy family as similar to what happens in a Twelve Step support group.[4]

It is intriguing to compare the parallels in Maddock and Manley's perceptions of healthy sexuality with the views of Native Americans. Sharon Day, writing about sexuality in the traditional peoples of North America, notes that women and men were equally valued and empowered. Their survival depended on that. Second, sexual diversity was not only tolerated but also honored. Gay and lesbian people were literally a third gender who were believed to have special healing gifts. All individuals were respected because every member of the tribe was important. Every adult honored and was active in the rearing of children. In many ways, these are the principles of the new paradigm described in chapter 1. An individual can effect a shift not only in his or her personal sexual paradigm, but also in the coming paradigm for all of us. [5]

For anorexics, a challenge exists. They have to make up the deficits of their own families and life experiences. They need a new "family" or clan or tribe to support them in these changes. It is almost like being reparented in order to reclaim their sexuality. They need to go through a whole relearning process with the help of new clan members and elders with a different covenant or contract about sexual issues. I call these new clan members and elders "fair witnesses."

Fair Witnesses

The concept of fair witnesses appeared first in a 1959 novel by Robert Heinlein called *Stranger in a Strange Land*. In this science fiction classic there was a class of government officials called "fair witnesses." These officials had infallible memories and were called on to witness any kind of contract from marriage to a business understanding. Trauma therapist Alice Miller borrowed the concept and applied it to trauma survivors. The idea was for victims to seek out witnesses who really knew what happened to them. These fair witnesses then could validate the victim's experience.

For example, I have a clinical associate who tells of a letter written by her grandfather. He had written it to his sister telling her of his concerns about how his granddaughter (my associate) was being treated. What he described is also what my associate remembered decades later. The letter is the only thing of her grandfather's that she has, and she treasures it. It confirms the abuse she remembered; it validates her perceptions of reality. It says she is not crazy.

A therapist can be a fair witness. After a session with a client's parents, the therapist might say to the client, "When your father teases you and tells you he is only joking, I do not believe that. He is being cruel and malicious." The therapist validates the client's experience. That is how the client felt, but the father was denying that reality. A fair witness is a person who can tell us the truth. This can be about the past or it can be about the present. I sometimes believe that people's mental health is directly related to the degree that they surround themselves with "truth-sayers." Mental health is a commitment to reality at all costs.

Because of the supercharged nature of talking about sexuality, recovering anorexics need to create a community of supportive people who will be honest with them. The healing process described in this book works best with fair witnesses. They can be

- a therapist
- a treatment group or therapeutic community
- a sponsor
- a trusted family member
- a trusted pastor
- friends
- fellow Twelve Step group members
- fellow anorexics

And, if we are in a relationship, our partner. I believe that in relationships we can make up for deficits. We can be nurtured by our partner without making him or her into a surrogate parent. Genuine nurturing by a loved one can go a long way to make up for past neglect and abuse.

Dimensions of Sexual Health

This book now presents a program for exploring your sexuality. The program is composed of twelve dimensions of sexual experience. These dimensions represent principles described earlier as the basic elements of the new paradigm: mutuality and equality; individual respect and dignity; commitment to nonabusive, nonviolent, and nonexploitive loving relationships that add meaning to life. These twelve dimensions are as follows.

Dimensions of Healthy Sexuality

1. NURTURING—the capacity to receive care from others and provide care for self.
2. SENSUALITY—the mindfulness of physical senses that creates emotional, intellectual, spiritual, and physical presence.
3. SELF-IMAGE—a positive self-perception that includes embracing your sexual self.
4. SELF-DEFINITION—a clear knowledge of yourself, both positive and negative, and the ability to express boundaries as well as needs.
5. COMFORT—the capacity to be at ease about sexual matters with oneself and with others.
6. KNOWLEDGE—a knowledge base about sex in general and about one's own unique sexual patterns.
7. RELATIONSHIP—a capacity to have intimacy and friendship with both those of the same gender and opposite gender.
8. PARTNERSHIP—the ability to maintain an interdependent, equal relationship that is intimate and erotic.
9. NONGENITAL SEX—the ability to express erotic desire emotionally and physically without the use of the genitals.
10. GENITAL SEX—the ability to freely express erotic feelings with the use of the genitals.
11. SPIRITUALITY—the ability to connect sexual desire and expression to the value and meaning of one's life.

12. Passion—the capacity to express deeply held feelings of desire and meaning about one's sexual self, relationships, and intimacy experience.

I described these dimensions in my book *Don't Call It Love.* At that time there were eight dimensions. Then I realized that what many professionals were describing as healthy sex matched the life principles of the Twelve Steps of Alcoholics Anonymous and related programs, and so I expanded the eight dimensions to twelve. Many recovering people of all varieties would ask me, "What is healthy sex?" I found that if they also applied Twelve Step principles to their sexuality, their sexual experience would be transformed. Moreover, integrating these principles into their sex lives would also cause healing in other areas of their lives. I soon concluded that this idea could probably help many people. Years of experience have now proven that this is true. And I know the Twelve Steps work for sexual anorexics. (A matrix is provided in appendix 1, which shows how the twelve dimensions of healthy sexuality match up and interrelate with twelve supportive strategies for changing our sexual paradigms and with the principles of the Twelve Steps.)

Each of the following chapters focuses on a specific dimension of sexual healing. Activities at the conclusion of each chapter help to foster that specific dimension of healthy sexuality in your life. Each chapter asks you to plan how you will enhance your sexuality over the next weeks and months using those activities. If you have a partner, the partner can be involved in this process. A set of self-assessment scales at the end of each chapter can be done separately or as couples. When you have completed all twelve chapters, you will also have clarified and defined a plan for yourself for an enduring and rewarding sexuality.

Here are some ways that people have used these materials:

- Couples have used the materials in meetings with therapists and supportive sponsors.
- Individuals have used the materials as part of their work in Twelve Step groups for sexual anorexia.
- Individuals have used the materials as part of a Twelve Step sharing group or accountability group.
- Individuals have simply used the material when talking with the people in their support network.
- Twelve Step groups in sexual-addiction recovery have used them as part of ongoing meetings and retreats.
- Couples groups such as Recovering Couples Anonymous have used the materials for a series of meetings on sexuality.
- Treatment facilities have used the materials as part of treatment, aftercare, and extended care.
- Couples groups, couples, and individuals not in recovery have used these materials.

There are many ways to use this process as long as you have the support and honesty of your fair witnesses along the way. Without such efforts, however, the second-order change will not occur.

There are some things I wish for you to remember as you proceed. First, you do not have to do this perfectly. To borrow a phrase that will be familiar to recovering people, "It is progress, not perfection, that counts." Second, reading the book alone will only be moderately helpful. Doing the exercises and sharing with your fair witnesses is where the real help will come. And, finally, when the going gets difficult and it feels like too much, remember that you do not do this simply for yourself. All of us need to be part of the paradigm shift. We need you. Do not give up. Not now.

PART
II

NURTURING

NURTURING—the ability and willingness to take care of ourselves and to accept care and kindness from others—is the absolute foundation upon which reclaiming and creating a healthy sexuality rests. Think of a gate that we can unlock and open. To be nurtured, we must first unlock and open ourselves to that possibility. However, if we have been living in and become comfortable with a life based on deprivation, unlocking and opening this gate can be very difficult. Accepting life as deprivation precludes an openness to nurturing. What's more, if we have difficulty nurturing ourselves or allowing others to do so, we will also have difficulty with sex. Deny nurturing, and we also deny our sexuality. Healthy sexuality is, by definition, nurturing—for both us and our partner.

Unfortunately, many of us have had little experience either with accepting nurturing or with nurturing ourselves; we may even have a hard time recognizing nurturing. Figure 6.1 offers some examples of ways to nurture ourselves and others.

RACHEL'S STORY

Rachel is the mother of four and a sexual anorexic. Before her marriage, she had a long history of repeatedly entering relationships in which men would exploit, degrade, and abuse her.

Over the years, Rachel "learned" that she was worthless and undeserving. She takes little care of herself, nor does she let others help or care for her. Instead, she lives to care for and meet the needs of her husband and children—they are her life. Rachel truly believes she is unworthy of a better life—or any life at all, for that matter.

Figure 6.1   Examples of Nurturing

Accepting Nurturing from Others	*Accepting Sexual Nurturing from Others*
• Allow someone to cook a special meal for you or take you to dinner. • Obtain help on a project for which you are responsible. • Go have a massage. • Let a therapist or physician help you. • Let a friend throw a party for you. • Let a friend take you to a movie.	• Accept compliments about your appearance and attractiveness. • Be willing to receive an erotic massage. • Ask for help on sexual matters. • Be willing to receive support from people of the same gender. • Allow your partner to orchestrate/prepare a sexual event. • Allow your partner to be supportive of you when facing sexual challenges. • Be willing to allow your partner to touch and massage your body.
Nurturing Yourself • Take a nap when you need one. • Listen to some favorite music. • Walk or sit by a lake or stream. • Save for and buy something you really want. • Do something to make your bed or bedroom more comfortable. • Seek out a favorite, peaceful place. • Fix a favorite meal. • Sleep in.	*Nurturing Yourself Sexually* • Buy and wear clothes that make you feel sexual and erotic. • Touch yourself in gentle, loving ways. • Ask for things that would be pleasurable for you. • Explore new ways to expand your sexual awareness.

Rachel's relationship with her husband is quite contentious. She finally sought therapy and treatment because, in the midst of one of their arguments, she hit him on the side of the head hard enough to break his eardrum. This incident so shocked her—she couldn't believe she had actually struck and injured her husband—that she finally realized how out of control she could get.

The pressures created by living only for others and taking no real care of oneself—living in deprivation, in other words—must be released somehow. In Rachel's case, it took the form of violence.

Despite living in such a desperate situation, Rachel had long put off therapy. She told herself she couldn't afford it. She had always avoided spending money on herself; everything she did, after all, was for her children. When she ultimately sought help, her intent was to come to therapy for only one week because she simply didn't feel she deserved any more help than that. Caring for herself simply isn't part of Rachel's life repertoire.

The Four Core Beliefs

As a child, Rachel, like so many people struggling with sexual anorexia and sexual addiction, learned a set of basic, or core, beliefs that are now central to her world as an adult. As described in chapter 2, each core belief contributes to the disconnection between the interior world she experiences with its pain and shame, and the exterior image she projects to keep her secret inner world safe.

The first of these four core beliefs—*I am basically a bad, unworthy person*—structures the emotional foundation of Rachel's world. As a child, Rachel's needs, desires, and accomplishments were regularly ignored or devalued, and from these experiences, she concluded that she was not a worthwhile person; feelings of inadequacy and failure, therefore, predominated. Unconsciously, she accepts humiliation and degradation as justified or deserved.

Rachel and others in similar predicaments are committed to hiding their inner reality from the world. To do so, they create a front of "normalcy" to disguise their profound sense of inadequacy. They may even appear grandiose and full of exaggerated self-importance. To the outside world, Rachel is the perfect, loving, self-sacrificing mother and spouse; on the inside, however, she suffers deeply. The front she has created stands in stark contrast to her self-defeating and degrading behavior.

The second belief—*No one could love me as I am*—also sustains the secret world. Rachel believes that everyone would abandon her if the truth about her were known. Consequently, she has a constant fear of being vulnerable or dependent on others. She perceives herself to be so bad that everything that goes wrong is her fault. She assumes responsibility for all the pain of her loved ones. Though she appears loving and kind, Rachel has ultimately become personally unreachable. The significant people in her life feel cut out, pushed away, useless, and neglected. This contradictory behavior is enormously confusing for them. How do they explain these feelings and the fact that she always seems to place their needs and wants first?

The third belief—*My needs are never going to be met if I have to depend on others*—provides the driving power for Rachel's life. Basically, Rachel feels unloved and unlovable, which means her needs will be unmet. The resulting rage (witness her violent outburst with her husband) has become internalized as depression, resentment, self-pity, and perhaps even suicidal feelings. This rage about past unmet needs prevents the possibility of her expressing needs now, because Rachel anticipates she will be rejected. Consequently, she appears not to want or need anything at a human level. Rachel is purposely unclear about her intentions in relationships, which creates a kind of seductive behavior; that is, she tries to be affirmed or cared for without expressing that she needs it—always to avoid rejection.

The final belief—*Sex is my most terrifying need*—creates the sexual anorexic's obsessive revulsion toward sex. (The sex addict's

Figure 6.2   The Core Beliefs and the Sexual Anorexic-Sexual Addiction Cycle

Sexual Anorexic   Sex Addict

Four Core beliefs	*Four Core beliefs*
1. I am basically a bad, unworthy person.	1. I am basically a bad, unworthy person.
2. No one could love me as I am.	2. No one could love me as I am.
3. My needs are never going to be met if I have to depend on others.	3. My needs are never going to be met if I have to depend upon others.
4. Sex is my most terrifying need.	4. Sex is my more important need.

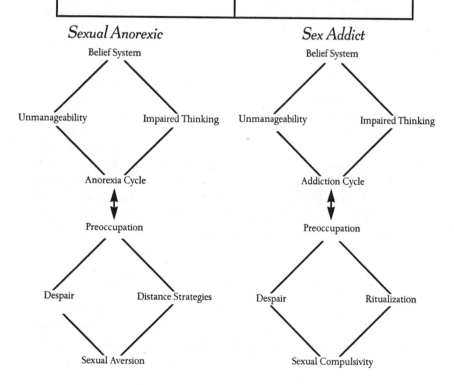

final core belief is just the opposite. It says, *Sex is my most important need.* Out of this need, then, comes the sex addict's compulsive sexual acting out.) Growing out of these core beliefs is a repeating cycle of self-deprivation—an obsessive habit with its own asceticism of sacrifice and providing for others. Figure 6.2 depicts the core beliefs and the sexual anorexic-sexual addiction cycle.

Nurturing—the ability and willingness to take care of ourselves and to accept care and kindness from others—is not only the absolute foundation on which reclaiming and creating a healthy sexuality rests; it also begins the dismantling of the four core beliefs. Nurturing demonstrates the lie of these beliefs. First, if someone, in fact, loves and cares for me, I cannot be unworthy of love and a bad person. Second, this person who loves me knows who I am—and yet still loves me. Third, I really do want to be nurtured and have my needs met, and here is a person who loves me and on whom I find myself depending for love and nurturing. Finally, as I begin to experience sexuality at its most basic level of nurturing, I find that it isn't as frightening as I had thought.

It's important to note once again that the illnesses of sexual anorexia, sexual bulimia, and sex addiction can be seen as a continuum of behaviors. Anorexics do have ways in which they act out, just as sex addicts do "act in" at times by denying themselves any sexual activity. Most people who have what is called sex addiction, in fact, fit in the middle category of sexual bulimia—flip-flopping between sexual bingeing and sexual denial. No one fits solely into one category, hence the concept of a continuum of behaviors (see figure 6.3).

Our Culture's "Antinurturing Curriculum"

We've now reached the crux of the dilemma. In order to be nurtured by someone or to nurture ourselves, we must have some sense that we are worthy of it, that we deserve it. A kind of "inner permission" for us to have nurturing must exist. Rachel desperately needs nurturing, but to let herself be nurtured goes against her most fundamental beliefs about herself as a person.

Rachel's struggle with nurturing is symptomatic of a broader societal problem—the existence of an "antinurturing curriculum." This curriculum teaches men to "tough-out" life, to sacrifice, to keep the upper lip stiff and not react emotionally (or at least not show any emotion), and to endure at all cost, and it teaches women to make their needs secondary to others at their own expense.

Women, however, may actually have an advantage over men when it comes to the ability to nurture and to accept nurturing because they are culturally encouraged to bond and nurture with others. They are taught that relationships are important, as are having and expressing feelings.

But women are caught in the cultural web too. Because of the power differentials between men and women in this culture, women are far more likely to be traumatized, victimized, and exploited. (As noted in chapter I, women in North America now have only a fifty-fifty chance of living their lives without being sexually assaulted.) Once we have been victimized or assaulted, we tend to view ourselves as somehow defective and not worth much. This, in turn, can damage our ability to accept

Figure 6.3   Continuum of Behaviors

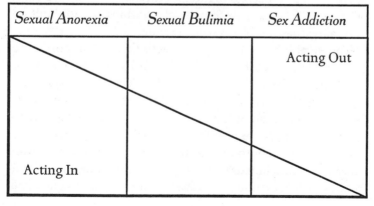

Sexual Anorexia	Sexual Bulimia	Sex Addiction
		Acting Out
Acting In		

ourselves, thus interfering with our ability to nurture and be nurtured.

Women are damaged, too, by simply growing up in this culture, one which systematically devalues and denies (both implicitly and explicitly) their worth as human beings. Women ultimately get the impression that they simply aren't worth the same as men—and not deserving of much—except when they are being pursued by men for a relationship.

Parenthetically, the devaluation of women is, I believe, why women have for so long been taught to hold back sex from men until they are married or, at the very least, believe they are in a committed, long-term relationship. Women sometimes, for example, have the experience of being sexual with a man whom they believe cares about them, only to find out the contrary. Here's the catch-22: It can be hard for women to know why a man is interested; does he just want sex, or does he really respect her as a person? It's a difficult double bind. A woman can be left to guess at the man's intentions because she won't know whether the man values her for more than sex until she has been sexual with him—and then if she finds he doesn't value her, it's too late. In a culture that devalues and denies power to women, some may decide to use sex as a way to reassert their power. What's happening here is that sex has become currency. Sex is "traded" for access to men's "currency"—money, power, prestige. As long as male-female relationships are not built on mutuality, these problems will continue.

Women also hear a message that tells them it's important to make their needs secondary to the needs of others in their lives—particularly their spouses and children—and this message opens the door to a life devoid of self-care or nurturing. Self-deprivation can become a way of life. This message reinforces the struggles of people like Rachel.

It's important not to underestimate how easily one can, over time, become acclimatized to such a life. I remember a time, for example, when I was sitting in therapy. My therapist's office had a window facing toward the sun, and as the sunlight streamed across the room, it hit me on the side of my face. To keep it out of my eyes, I started to arch my face and my neck. By the time we had neared the end of the session, I was leaning over the left side of my chair in an incredibly awkward position.

At this point, my therapist said, "Pat, please. Stop now. Move your chair. I just wanted to see how long you would go on with this. Are you aware that you were so focused, so task oriented, that you've made yourself extremely uncomfortable? Had you checked in on yourself for just a second, you couldn't have failed to notice your discomfort. All you needed to do was move your chair about two feet to your right, and you wouldn't have had the sun in your eyes at all."

I was shocked at the time at how focused outside of myself I was at that moment and I saw how I did that in other parts of my life too. I would neglect my own self-comfort and not attend to my own needs, in part, because in my family, I learned how to tolerate discomfort and not attend to my own needs. All of us do this to some extent, but not to the extent that those of us who've lived in neglectful families do so.

The Effects of Neglect

If children are neglected, if their fundamental nurturing and survival needs are not attended to, they will not learn how to take care of themselves. Thus childhood neglect can also feed into later problems with lack of nurturing from within and without, various types of deprivation, and sexual anorexia.

Let me share another example. Jake grew up in a rural area during World War II. His father was in Europe, leaving his mother to tend the farm. As a result, neither Jake nor his siblings received much attention, not out of maliciousness, but because there simply wasn't enough time to go around.

In such circumstances, Jake had lots of time to himself and frequently got himself into bad situations. Jake didn't know how to take care of himself because no adult had showed him how to do so *by taking care of him.* Jake eventually learned that the only way he could start to feel better was to take responsibility for himself. If he didn't, no one would. No one was going to help him stay out of trouble. But this situation also left him feeling that somehow he didn't deserve to be taken care of. He wasn't good enough or worthy enough to merit the care he wanted and needed.

Another potential response to neglect—the other end of the continuum, if you will—are feelings of "entitlement." "Entitled" adults believe they simply deserve whatever they want. Life owes them! They expect others to know what they want, what they're thinking, what they need.

This belief can have two causes. First, as children, they may have never been taken care of, and thus never learned self-care. The core of their problem lies, then, in the reality that they never learned how to ask for nurturing or even that nurturing was an option for them. The result is often that they never learn how to appropriately take care of themselves. They just wait for it, expecting whatever they are to get to come from someone else. The other cause of entitlement beliefs is excessive care. When parents do so much for their children, giving them everything they want, children never learn to do much for themselves. Once they grow up and get out into the world, they have no self-care skills. They don't know how to nurture others, either, but they are more than happy to accept care *from* others. Again, they believe that they are simply *entitled* to it. In addition, the overly nurtured child actually experiences a high degree of invasion from the parents, which results in difficulties with boundaries later in life. The child never learns how to self-protect by saying, for example, "No, I don't want to do that" or, "No, I don't need that" because the parents continually do whatever they want for (or to) the child.

Interestingly, children from some homes may exhibit this sense of entitlement as a result of both neglect and excessive care. On the one hand, all their material needs and wants may be taken care of without effort on their part. On the other hand, they are often denied emotional bonding and modeling from adults. This is due both to cultural imperatives such as reserve, decorum, and formality, and to being raised by professional caregivers.

An excellent source of additional information on the issues of entitlement and neglect is the book *Emotional Incest Syndrome* by Patricia Love. Love describes how problems with neglect and entitlement can occur even within the same family. In such cases, one child is chosen as the "special" one, while others are neglected. Both have problems as a result, but for opposite reasons.

Whether deprived, neglected, or entitled, or a combination of the three, the result is the same. These people know neither how to care for themselves nor how to ask for help. There's an old Al-Anon joke about how to recognize a person who grew up in a dysfunctional family. When the person goes to the grocery store to buy just one item and can't find it, rather than ask where it is, he or she walks up and down the aisles until the item is finally found—wasting a lot of time and effort in the process. For most people, it's *fine* to ask for help. Most of us would say that, of course, it's okay for someone to help us by telling us that the paprika's in aisle seven! This is just a small act of nurturing. But consider this: If we can't even ask someone where the paprika is, how are we going to tell our partner what we need to meet our sexual needs?

When I'm working with a client and I really want to figure out what's going on with the client's family, I ask how help was given. The answer to this simple question reveals volumes about that past and present. In my own family, for example, when I asked for help, I received it—but only with a lecture on the fact that if I had to ask for help, it's because I didn't do something right in the first place. If whatever it was had been done right, I was told, I wouldn't have needed to ask. Eventually, of course, I simply quit asking.

A patient of mine, whom I'll call "Jim," described a different but equally destructive pattern from his childhood.

This situation happened with regularity. I'd have a school project, for example, which I needed help to complete. I'd go to my parents well in advance of the deadline and ask for help. "We'll work on it Saturday," they would say. But when Saturday arrived, something would come up. They couldn't help, but they'd say, "We'll get to it Sunday night." But Sunday night, something else would get in the way, and help was put off until the next weekend. But that weekend, they were going out of town. "But that's okay," I was told. "We'll get to it. Don't worry, we've got a week left to work on this." The next plan was to work on the project Monday night, but then the boss asked Dad to work late and Mom said she was too busy. Finally, it's Wednesday night, the project is due Friday, and this act has been playing out for nearly four weeks. I'm desperate for help, but my parents shout, "Why did you wait until the last minute? You could have been working on this all this time. Now it's going to be a lot of trouble for everyone. We have to drop everything to help you, and everyone else has to suffer because of your bad planning."

Over the years, what lesson did Jim learn? That asking for help means getting himself into trouble, and, worse yet, he won't really get the help he needs, either. In addition, Jim decided it doesn't make sense to ask for help from or trust people who are close to him.

If we can't trust others, including a partner, sex just won't work—*unless* we make the other person into an object, which leads to a difficult relationship at best, if not to addiction, as we'll see.

Objectification of Others

When we're asking for help, we're open, emotionally vulnerable, and dependent on another person. Rejection is an ever-present possibility. If, however, we view others as objects, we can't be rejected. We're in control of the situation, and we don't have to depend on that "object" for anything. And, most important, we're not emotionally vulnerable.

Parenthetically, this is how we teach people to be addicts.

When we grow up in families in which others do not follow through for us, we learn not to trust anyone. And if we can't trust that other people will give us what we need, then we start looking for things we can trust—and one thing about alcohol, sex, food, gambling, high-risk behavior, and so on is that they deliver (but only to a point, of course!). Addiction, seen this way, is a pathological relationship with a mood-altering experience.

In healthy relationships, those involved relate to *each other*. This is how we learn to be interdependent. In addictive relationships, people relate to an experience—the drug high, the hustle, the sex act. Even if another human being is involved, as in prostitution, for example, the other person is objectified, is not seen as a person. There are no demands. You just put your money on the table, get what you came for, and walk out the door.

Healthy sex requires a fundamental relationship transaction. Going through the physiological responses with a prostitute, for example, might make you feel better temporarily, but it won't ever satisfy the deeper soul needs for intimacy and bonding. In many ways, addiction can be characterized as the failure to bond.

Healthy Sexuality Requires Letting Go

In addition to believing we are worthy of being nurtured, healthy sexuality requires that we also have the willingness and ability to "let go"—to be open to nurturing. Letting go requires giving up control. Survivors of trauma—those who grew up in homes in which chemical, physical, or emotional abuse existed—regularly experienced circumstances where their level of anxiety was very high. Everyone learned that it wasn't safe to trust others. Because life was so random and chaotic, the "solution" that members of such families usually turn to is trying to control as much around them as possible. The need to control can also grow in rigid and rule-oriented families. When we learn as children to try to control all our circumstances and interactions with others, it's natural to simply carry this approach into our adult lives and relationships.

When we as children don't feel nurtured, we live with a high level of anxiety, and one response to anxiety is the attempt to control. This is what neglect does to children. As we have seen, a family can be both rigid and neglectful. Being taken care *of* doesn't guarantee being cared *for*—emotional support can be missing.

Growing up in an emotionally abusive and neglectful family, Rachel learned to do whatever she could to control her environment to get what she needed. Maintaining constant attempts to control all situations and others in our lives to get what we need, however, precludes receiving nurturing. Controlling and nurturing are mutually exclusive, as Rachel's life exemplifies so well.

Healthy sex is possible only when we are well disposed to doing good things for ourselves and to letting other people do good things for us. Healthy sex requires letting go of ourselves, of allowing touch and feeling, of responding to and giving to others. If we've lived for years unable to accept nurturing from others or ourselves, there's simply no magic switch that will engage the ability to nurture and be nurtured that is required for healthy sex. If we can't give up control, we can't allow ourselves to surrender to this process of change.

Deeply entrenched core beliefs can't be overridden instantaneously, however. Saying so won't make it so; instead, we need self-awareness to understand what's happening, and a good deal of work to make the needed changes.

Nurturing as a Step One Issue

Most sexual anorexics with whom I've worked find that the healing journey begins when they acknowledge that they have a problem and that their lives have become unmanageable as a result of it. This is the First Step of all Twelve Step programs.

The first act of opening, of vulnerability, is to acknowledge the problem. By so doing, we are asking for help and allowing other people into our lives. We are opening to the possibility of a relationship. But to do so also requires us to admit that we are in pain, to admit just how badly we are hurting. Of course, this can be very difficult, and particularly so for people who have been living in deprivation. But opening to and entering into this pain, regardless of the outcome, is the only way to finally leave it behind.

To better explain how meaning and growth can come out of facing one's suffering, let me offer several examples. Many traditional cultures require all boys to pass through an initiation rite before they can be accepted as men by their society. These adolescents grow up in cultures that meet their needs differently than our culture meets the needs of adolescents. A larger group of adults (often belonging to the extended family) is responsible for raising and caring for children and adolescents, thus increasing the chances that at any given time, some adult will be present for the child. Children are supported not just by their nuclear families, but by all members of the society, clan, or tribe.

These cultures assume that life will bring challenges. To prepare young men well for adulthood, they have to be put in a different situation from what they expected—the initiation. Elders from a different clan carry out the initiation. They are the youths' spiritual directors, guiding them through the pain of initiation while helping them understand, in part, that they will experience pain in their adult lives. And, since that pain is unavoidable, the elders teach these young men how to handle it. They give the youth the spiritual direction, skills, and support they will need to go through painful moments. And because their guides are elders they do not know, the initiates learn that they can be cared for by adults whom they do not know. These young men, when called by the elders, fear the passage. They don't want to go, but they have no choice; they surrender to the process. They find comfort in knowing that others have preceded them and have survived to become men.

Literature and myth are replete with tales of heroes and heroines called to a challenge. Initially, none want to accept it or to enter into suffering. All are afraid. They make excuses. But ultimately they do accept the challenge and then set out on the journey. On the path, they discover help when it is needed, often from a master or an elder, and eventually they overcome their pain and suffering.

Joseph Campbell writes extensively about facing one's suffering in his book *Hero with a Thousand Faces*. It is the journey of all heroes and heroines. It is the journey of Everyman and Everywoman. This may be your journey too. You may be reading this book not because you want to, but because you are on a healing journey. What I am suggesting you do is to trust yourself and to seek out "new elders" who can help—your *fair witnesses*. I am saying "Let help in" because it's not possible to travel this journey alone. We need our new elders, our groups, our fair witnesses for support.

Sexual anorexics literally have to surrender to the pain of their emptiness and incompleteness, to experience first the pain and then the transformation, which go with surrender and suffering. Admitting and accepting the pain we have been living in will enable us to ultimately rise above it, to shed the need for it, and to become a healthier adult. This giving over to suffering allows us to be at long last nurtured. When we accept this challenge, we will find the help we need to succeed. Opening to suffering becomes a means of transformation through which it is possible to become more than we ever before imagined.

KEY QUESTIONS

In workshops and in my counseling experience, the following questions come up regularly in reference to nurturing.

> *If sex is an activity for adults, how do I nurture the child within about sex?*

This question is often raised because one of the ways to abuse children is to prematurely expose them to adult sexuality. When we are nurturing this child within, it is important that we be sensitive to past experiences and the feelings that we carry as a result, so that we don't overwhelm the inner child with our adult sexual concerns.

Remember, first, that we are always sexual people—even when we're children. Next, recognize that it is the adult's task to keep the child safe while doing inner-child work.

Again, however, we must return to what is *the* fundamental issue: What most affects adult sexuality is the inability to accept care and nurture—an inability that is *learned*. We are working to recreate a general acceptance of nurturing that flows out of childlike openness—while still remembering that we are adults who must ensure our safety. We need to trust ourselves, which requires good judgment—something we will look into more in the next chapters—because as we move into more overtly sexual tasks, we will have to feel that our inner child is safe.

Even though the care and nurturing we are talking about at this time are neither overtly sexual nor erotic, they will create a solid platform on which we can build a healthy adult sexuality. We will see that our First Step is to admit we have a need for nurturing—in general, not just sexually— and to allow it into our lives. Over and over and over again I see people who want to rush into working on sexual techniques, so I can't overemphasize the need to build a foundation in nurturing first. The fundamental building block of healthy sexuality is the ability to be nurtured, to feel comfortable with being nurtured, to give ourselves over to being nurtured. If we can't do this, it will never be possible, as an adult, to have healthy sex.

Everybody says to nurture yourself, but I don't know how to do that or what it feels like.

Some people may find it hard to believe that an individual might not know how to self-nurture, but hearing this question as I often do, there's no doubt that this is a great struggle for many.

At the end of this chapter are exercises designed to help people begin to learn to nurture themselves and accept nurturing from others. One suggestion I have now, however, is to be serious about nurturing, but not too solemn. What's the distinction between the two? Watch a child working on a project; building a fort, for instance. Kids can work for hours on something like this and be quite serious about it. Yet at the same time they will play and laugh and giggle. They're serious, but not solemn.

Too often, however, we as adults will not let go enough to be serious and playful. We become stuck in solemnity. When the question is asked about the difference between the two, it's asked with solemnity. We want to do everything correctly, properly.

When we are depleted, we need to allow ourselves room to grow, so my suggestion is to accept that we don't really know how to be nurtured, that we have to learn, and that we can learn. Next, just be open to the possibility of nurturance. Once open to the possibility, we will experience it. And that experience may come almost as a revelation, wherein suddenly we will see the myriad possibilities for nurturing in our lives.

When is sex a fix and when is it nurturing?

This question is often asked by sex addicts, as well as by alcoholics and those with other addictions. Their concern is that they always used sex as a kind of medicating tool. Consequently, when they have sexual feelings they think, "Oh, no, I must be needing to medicate, and this is addictive behavior," even though they could very well be having quite normal feelings of arousal appropriate to the situation.

In early recovery, sex addicts often bounce from the addiction side of their problem to the anorexic side. They are still obsessed with sexual issues; now, however, on the anorexic side of the equation, they believe that total abstinence is the only solution.

Here are some guidelines to help determine whether sex is appropriate—and SAFE, a formula recovering people have used for many years now.

- Sex is safe when it isn't Secret.
- Sex is safe when it isn't Abusive.
- Sex is safe when it isn't something we do just because we Feel bad about something.
- Sex is safe when it's not Empty of relationship.

In addition, sex is safe when

- it doesn't feel shameful
- it doesn't demean others
- it's celebrative

An additional suggestion: Whenever you're in doubt, check with somebody you trust and get another opinion. This could be your sponsor, your therapist, or one of your fair witnesses, for example. Remember, too, that as time passes, you'll grow in your recovery and have a better sense of addictive sex and nurturing sex. Figure 6.4 summarizes the differences between addictive and healthy sexuality.

ISSUES

When working on nurturing skills, many sexual anorexics struggle with issues such as the following. Some of these issues have been explored at greater length in this or previous chapters; for those which have not, a brief discussion is included here. Read the issues carefully, noting the ones that apply to you. Then use those issues as discussion points with your partner and/or fair witnesses.

❋ Avoiding extremes of indulgence and deprivation.
While we looked at this topic in depth in chapter 3, remember that it is very easy to find ourselves living in extremes. It is so important to seek out the center in our lives, and one of the ways we can stay in balance is to connect with ourselves, with our inner voice and core. When we do so, we finally begin to know who we are and what we want. To know ourselves, we have to let go and really look at and address our problems, which is what this book is designed to help us do.

❋ Feeling unworthy or undeserving of care.
This issue has to do with shame. Psychoanalyst Erik Erikson, many years ago, talked about the eight stages of human development. In the first stage, the baby must decide whether or not to trust its caregiver—a most basic feeling.

Following this stage comes "shame versus autonomy." In this stage, the child begins to "leave" the parent to take independent action. The child needs to be assured that the parent will still be there for her, but she begins to learn to be on her own, make choices for herself, and take responsibility for herself. If there is failure to accomplish this stage, the child feels shame. Eventually, such children lose the ability to be individuals, to act proactively for themselves. When they grow into adulthood, they find themselves with little or no sense of self and profound feelings of shame—with the door wide open for addictive behaviors to fill that empty place inside them. We hear them as adults, after they have begun to recover, asking why they can't drink, for example, but other people can. Or why they can't eat and enjoy their food as others can. Or why sex is such a problem for them. They feel flawed, ashamed. If we feel flawed and shameful, we don't believe we deserve anything good—and now we're back to the need to learn nurturing.

❋ Having difficulty separating care from exploitation or abandonment.

Figure 6.4

Addictive Sexuality	Healthy Sexuality
• Feels shameful	• Adds to self-esteem
• Is illicit, stolen, or exploitive	• Has no victims
• Compromises values	• Deepens meaning
• Draws on fear for excitement	• Uses vulnerability for excitement
• Reenacts childhood abuses	
• Disconnects one from oneself	• Cultivates sense of being adult
• Creates a world of unreality	• Furthers sense of self
• Is self-destructive and dangerous	• Expands reality
• Uses conquest or power	• Relies on safety
• Serves to medicate and kill pain	• Is mutual and intimate
• Is dishonest	• Takes responsibility for needs
• Becomes routine	• May bring legitimate suffering
• Requires a double life	• Originates in integrity
• Is grim and joyless	• Presents challenges
• Demands perfection	• Integrates most authentic parts of self
	• Is fun and playful
	• Accepts the imperfect

Two basic points need to be reiterated here, the first of which has to do with how help is given in the family and how care is accepted. In abusive families, children learn that care comes with a price—and often that price is exploitation. The child is told, "I'm doing this for you," or he somehow receives the message that help and care are being given to meet the child's needs. But, in fact, the opposite is true; the "caregivers" are really only meeting their own needs. The conclusion the child eventually reaches is that in order to get his needs met, he has to deny his own reality—lie, in other words—or do things that he knows are not right or good for him. The end result: distrust of any form of care.

The second point deals with the problem of abandonment.

People who've experienced significant abandonment during childhood may decide as adults that any relationship is better than another abandonment. Sexual abuse. Emotional abuse. Beatings. Emotional blackmail. Anything is acceptable, just not abandonment.

Most children grow up experiencing disappointments and a few "black eyes." But they learn, in general, that it's safe to trust themselves and others—that the world is a safe place. For people who've experienced severe abuse, however, care has always been contaminated with exploitation or abandonment. As a result, the freewheeling, open-hearted trust that is the child's natural stance in the world is destroyed. As children, these people learned to shut down. And as adults, they face the challenge of discovering that they can be nurtured and cared for *without* being exploited or left.

Furthermore, at this crucial juncture the First Step becomes very important. The first thing we need to do is to set our anxiety aside and allow the program laid out in this book to help. We are asked to trust the process of change. We learn that people work through the Steps and by so doing, they heal. Their needs are met—and the gate described in the first paragraph of this chapter begins to open.

✾ Overcoming rules about hardship and character building. As children, some of us learned certain rules about hardship. We learned that life was simply about suffering and that we have to accept it; that our body is bad; that we have to work until we're completely depleted; that we don't accept or even expect joy in our lives. Working hard on dismal and focused tasks without joy has become the central theme for us. Garrison Keillor, host of National Public Radio's *A Prairie Home Companion*, captures this attitude wonderfully when he describes the "Norwegian Bachelor Farmer" who isn't married, has few friends, and lives as independently as possible. Embedded in this caricature are our rules about accepting hardship and deprivation.

We can discover the childhood messages about hardship that prevent us today from being spontaneous and joyful and passionate. We can decide to make new rules for our lives and allow ourselves celebration, passion, and joy.

❋ Granting permission for sexuality to be nurturing and playful.
When children grow up in restrictive and nonnurturing environments, they lose their sense of playfulness and optimism. In addition, they develop a kind of attitude about their families that tells them they're being disloyal if they go against what they've been taught about nurturing, spontaneity, or playfulness. And here is another situation in which our "new elders"—our fair witnesses—can play a critical role in recovery. These people can give us permission to break these old rules and live in a way that is more fully human.

❋ Confronting blocks in the form of perfectionism, excessive goal orientation, and dependency avoidance.
Playfulness, spontaneity, nurturing, fun—all these and more are part of a healthy life. Author Berry Sears, in his best-selling book *The Zone*, talks at length about learning to "eat in the zone" by balancing proteins and carbohydrates and fats, and so on. In a similar way, we need to learn to live in the "healthy human zone"—a place where it's acceptable to make mistakes, to be playful . . . and to be sexual. We have had blocks that have kept us from living in the human zone; only by confronting them can we find our way back to it.

The following story illustrates well the consequences of a life lived without nurturing.

SEAN AND MARGIT

Sean and his wife, Margit, had been professionally trained and earned professional salaries when they were married in 1970.

Sean and Margit were also a product of their times—very counterculture—and so they were determined not to be part of, in Sean's words, "the exploitive, capitalistic world." As part of their wedding vows, they thus agreed to spend no more on themselves than the amount of money the federal government determined was the poverty level. The rest of their money would be donated to worthy causes. In addition, they chose to live in a commune.

As the years passed, Sean and Margit held rigorously to their goal, pinching pennies and living extremely frugally. They were dedicated to social causes and financially supported them as best they could. They were, however, also living in deprivation in the broader sense described in this book. What's more, Sean had been acting out sexually, and in quite dangerous ways.

Sean, fortunately, sought help and joined a Sex Addicts Anonymous (SAA) program. Though he came each week to meetings, he found it very difficult to stop his behavior. All along, the group posed a question commonly asked when members have relapsed. The group said, "What are you doing to take care of yourself?" As the group regularly wrestled with Sean about the concept of taking care of himself, it became more and more apparent that he didn't know what this meant. Under the regimen that he and his wife lived, he simply didn't take care of himself or his needs; he didn't do much at all that was nice for himself.

Finally one night, the group got on him, asking, "Sean, what's something that you've always wanted that you have never felt you could have or deserve?" And out of his mouth it popped. A Pendleton wool shirt. "I know it seems so frivolous to buy a name-brand shirt," he immediately added, "and I don't really need one. But I've always kind of wanted one."

That night, after the meeting, the group took Sean to a men's clothing store in a nearby shopping mall and stood there while he bought himself a Pendleton shirt! At long, long last, Sean had broken his rule about living in deprivation. The ultimate result? Sean and Margit now live in a nice home on a lake in a large metro area. They set aside 10 percent of their incomes for charitable organizations, but they travel, go out to eat, and generally enjoy themselves. And Sean hasn't acted out sexually in fifteen years.

Sean's experience demonstrates how deprivation and compulsion are related. If we live in deprivation, our lives will be out of control somewhere—and again, the most basic antidote to deprivation is to be good to ourselves.

TASKS

For many people who have abused alcohol or other drugs, the answer is sobriety through abstinence. Likewise, many people struggle with sexual anorexia because they've been out of control sexually. But in this case, abstinence is not the answer; it is instead just one more way of self-abuse, of failure to nurture, of self-deprivation.

The fundamental antidote for deprivation is the ability to nurture ourselves. Before we can have healthy, fulfilling sexual relationships, we must first learn how to let go and accept being nurtured by ourselves or by others.

The following exercises can help you begin this process. They offer concrete and specific ways to accept nurturing and allow yourself to depend on others. In addition, they will help you see how this lack of nurturing in your life has affected your sexual life.

ROLES AND RULES

People can take on any number of roles in their lives—some of which include
- the super-functional rescuer who has no time for self
- the martyr who has been well trained and well rewarded for tolerating pain
- the super-successful professional or business person on whom everyone depends to keep things going

- the "entitled" person who waits for others to take care of his or her needs, and then feels disappointed when nobody does so
- the hardworking underachiever who is burdened on all fronts, and who doesn't seem to be able to get ahead—who works very hard and yet has no reward in the end

NOW THINK ABOUT YOUR LIFE:

1. What roles have you played that interfered with being nurtured?

2. What roles have you played that interfered with taking care of yourself?

   Write your answers in your journal. (See "In Your Journal," page 123.)

AGAIN, THINK ABOUT YOUR LIFE:

3. Can you discover the messages about hardship that you learned as a child—messages that currently prevent you from being spontaneous and joyful and passionate? List these messages in your journal.

4. You can decide to make new rules for your life. In your journal, write new rules that will allow you to be spontaneous and joyful and passionate.

NURTURING YOURSELF

1. There are many ways we can nurture and care for ourselves. In this exercise, take some time to look carefully at yourself and try to discover ways you have *not* cared for yourself. Write your answers in your journal.

2. Now, do the opposite. What are some ways you *are* being good to yourself? In what ways do you reward yourself? If

you find this difficult at first, think of people you know who seem to be good at self-nurturing, and write down how you think they do it; also, refer to the nurturing chart at the beginning of this chapter. List your answers in your journal.

3. What are some additional ways you could nurture yourself?[7]

4. Turn now to the sexual part of your life. List ways you have been depriving yourself sexually or have kept yourself from being sexual.

5. Look at the list you just made about ways you have avoided being sexual. How have these choices hurt you—and others in your life? List your answers in your journal.

6. What has been painful about this exercise?

7. What are some ways you *could* nurture yourself sexually?

Again, if you have difficulty nurturing yourself or allowing others to do so, you will also have difficulty with sex. Deny nurturing, and you will also deny your sexuality. Again, healthy sexuality is, by definition, nurturing—for both you *and* your partner.

PLANNING

In this planning section, as well as those in the following chapters, you will make a plan of action to carry out the tasks of the previous section.

In the exercises in the tasks section, you were asked (1) to write some new rules for your life that will allow you to be more spontaneous, joyful, and passionate; and (2) to list ways you could nurture yourself, both in general and sexually.

Decide now how and when you will do this. Look at your

lists and choose two or three areas on which you will act during the next week or two. As you become more comfortable with nurturing yourself, return to your lists and add those nurturing activities to your life too.

You may also find yourself thinking of more new ways to nurture yourself. Add these to your lists and incorporate them into your life, too, as you feel comfortable doing so.

To further open yourself to nurturing and sensuality, I want to recommend a simply wonderful book of poetry, *Passionate Hearts*, by Wendy Maltz. Buy it or borrow it from the library, and then read and talk about one poem each day with your partner.

IN YOUR JOURNAL

As you progress through the self-help part of this book, you will experience many changes. One way to keep track of where we are—and where we've been—is to write our thoughts in a journal. This and later chapters suggest various journal exercises that you will find very useful and that will support your growth in healthier relationships and in your sexuality. For your journal, consider buying one of the many "blank books" available in most bookstores. If you currently have a spouse or partner, encourage him or her to keep such a journal too.

In *The Artist's Way*, a wonderful book about breaking through our creative blocks, Julia Cameron suggests creating "daily pages" in a journal. We can adapt her idea to breaking through our blocks related to nurturing. Begin each morning by filling about three pages with all the thoughts that come to you. Don't worry about organizing them or monitoring them. Just write them down! Write until you're spent—which will likely take fifteen or twenty minutes. Journal writing, or journaling, will help you get past your mind's surface chatter to what you are really thinking and feeling on a given morning. By so doing, you can better connect with your creativity.

FOCUS ON NURTURING

Since this chapter focuses on nurturing, also pay attention to ways you nurture yourself (or avoid it) each day and write them in your journal. At the end of each day, you and your partner could share what you've written.

A CLOSING EXERCISE

✐ Chapter 6 through chapter 17 close with an exercise that asks you and your partner to evaluate yourselves and one another on the chapter's focus. The closing exercise offers a wonderful opportunity for you to discover your strengths and weaknesses, as well as a chance for you and your partner to compare your perceptions of yourselves and one another. Over the course of chapters 6 through 17, these exercises will also help you chart your progress in building a healthy sexuality.

In addition to filling out the rating scales, it will be helpful to do the following:

- Once you have filled out your scales, share the results with your fair witnesses.
- After your partner has finished, talk about your partner's perceptions too. They may differ from yours and/or those of your fair witnesses.
- If significant discrepancies exist, note them and then return to your fair witnesses to look into them more carefully.

As you work on these scales, try not to become defensive if the perceptions your partner or your fair witnesses have of you differ from your own perceptions of yourself. Let these differences—and the reasons for them—be a source of information for all of you.

If you are not currently in a relationship, ask one of your fair witnesses (therapist, sponsor, anorexia group member, Twelve Step support group member, or RCA group member, for example) to work through the scales with you.

Part 1: Focus on You

Consider nurturing as it applies to you. Are you able to nurture yourself? Are you able to nurture others? How much work do you need on nurturing to feel comfortable with your skills?

Circle your rating on the scale below. (1 = low skills, need much work; 10 = high skills, need no further work.)

Next, ask your partner to think about your nurturing skills. On the same scale below, have your partner use a square to rate you.

1   2   3   4   5   6   7   8   9   10

Part 2: Focus on Your Partner

On this second scale, ask your partner to consider his or her own nurturing skills and ability. Is your partner able to self-nurture? To nurture others? How much work does your partner need to feel comfortable with his or her skills?

Have your partner use a circle to rate himself or herself.

Next, you rate your partner's nurturing ability. Use a square to do so.

1   2   3   4   5   6   7   8   9   10

Nurturing

Nurturing—
We learn to trust and to open our lives to experience.

SENSUALITY

These are our first real experiences of life—floating in a warm liquid, curling inside a total embrace, swaying to the undulations of the moving body, and hearing the beat of a pulsing heart.

—Desmond Morris

BEFORE YOU BEGIN reading this chapter, stop for a few moments. Close your eyes, take a few deep, slow breaths, and begin paying attention to your senses.

What sounds do you hear around you—the hum of a fan, someone talking in another room, a radio playing? What smells are floating in the air—food, perfume, flowers, the morning dew? What can you feel? The clothes on your body, the pressure of the chair you're sitting in, your glasses resting on your nose? Are there any flavors you can taste?

Were you a bit surprised at all that you were able to sense? Did you realize that so much was happening around you, that your body was giving you so much information? If you didn't, you're by no means unusual. In our culture, many people tune out much of what they're sensing. We're generally so focused on the task at hand—or what we forgot to do or have yet to accomplish—that we miss most of what's happening around us.

Mark Schwartz, a colleague of mine who has written and

lectured extensively on human sexuality, spent the early years in his career working with the internationally acclaimed human sexuality researchers William Masters and Virginia Johnson. Schwartz often talks about how Masters, Johnson, and the other early researchers were truly amazed by the number of physiological changes that occur during sexual arousal—changes that often pass totally unnoticed by most of us. If in everyday life we are not aware of what we are hearing, seeing, feeling, smelling, and tasting—of what we are perceiving in the broadest sense of the word—we won't notice what we're perceiving during sex, either. We simply miss these marvelous feelings and sensations. No magic switch for turning on our senses exists.

The Natural Sensuality of Children

To learn more about sensuality, we need only pay attention to children. Their ability to see and feel the world in unique ways is unceasingly amazing. A story from my own life illustrates this well.

One of my daughters, Erin, and her friend, Kelly, helped me open to another area of sensuality I'd never before considered. I had picked them up from soccer practice, and on the way to Kelly's house, the two of them, sitting in the backseat of the car, were planning what they were going to wear to the pool the next day—right down to the exact color of their shorts. As I listened to their conversation (kids just forget adults are present sometimes!), I was truly astounded by the depth and sophistication with which these two little girls were thinking about their clothing.

After dropping Kelly off at her home, I said to Erin, "You know, boys don't talk like that about clothes." She looked at me and said, "Why not?" Her reply really caught me off guard. I just didn't have a good answer.

When I got home that night, however, on a whim I decided to call my friend Warren and ask him what he was going to wear the next day. Warren's a quick study, and he picked up on this right away, replying, "Well, I'm going to wear my blue blazer and my regimental tie." To which I replied, "Oh, Warren, I love you in that." Warren then proceeded to call all our male friends to see what *they* were going to wear the next day. We had a blast with this!

We men don't generally think about our clothes. We don't think about colors or textures—the sensuality of these things. But it can be fun to do this. Certain clothes *do* feel and look good on our bodies.

Paying Attention to Senses

Have you ever taken a bit of time—an hour, half an hour, or even ten minutes—just to pay attention to what's around you? Before you continue reading, again put down this book and walk to the nearest window. Take five or ten minutes, or however long you want, to really look, to see, the colors and shapes of the world outside.

What did you notice that you'd never seen before? Remarkable, isn't it? Not long ago, for example, while driving to work, I saw a kind of woodpecker known as a red-breasted sapsucker only four feet from my car. I stopped and just stared at it. With its fluffy large red head, it was gorgeous! There was a time in my life when I would never have noticed that bird, and, even if I had, I'd never have stopped to watch it.

Perhaps what so many people find attractive and rewarding about being in natural settings is that it reawakens their sensuality. Away from the bustle and buzz of urban life, sounds and sights and smells flood our senses. I know when I hunt or fish, or otherwise spend time out of doors, I'm far more aware of my surroundings—the weather and temperature, for example—as well as of my body. When I return to my home in the city, I find I'm able to maintain this heightened awareness for a while, but soon I again become caught up in activities and focus primarily on how much I have to do. I don't notice the sky anymore, or the weather or the trees. *Not noticing* is the crux of this issue. Our bodies are always open to sensory input, but we aren't aware of it because, for any number of reasons, we simply don't pay attention.

Sensuality and Spirituality

Sensuousness requires stopping and paying attention. Once we do this, a new, deeper realm of experiences will open before us. Many religious and spiritual traditions recognize and acknowledge the connection between sensuality and spirituality. By truly opening to all that our senses bring us, we can become more open to and aware of the world around us—and thus we see the magnificence of creation. And marveling at its existence, we ask ourselves how all that is around us came to be. Native American traditions view sexuality differently than Western cultures, stemming in part, as discussed in chapter 5, from a close connection to and spiritually based respect for the surrounding world.

Many religious traditions also acknowledge that the beginning of a spiritual life starts with marveling, with this sense of wonder about creation. When people are asked where they feel most spiritual, far and away the most common response is that it's in a natural setting.

Our senses allow this marveling to happen. Nurturing opens the gate a crack, and sensuality pushes it open wide. When we are in natural settings, we are generally not focused on the past or the future. We're not focused on goals. We're not focused on work. Anxiety begins to drop away. We see and feel and touch and smell and hear creation. We perceive it. We marvel at it. We are struck, then, with a feeling of profound wonder. Could it be that there is more to life that we thought?

We begin to realize that not only is this world beautiful and amazing, but also it has a purpose and meaning—and because we are part of this creation, so do our lives likewise have purpose and meaning. We soon find ourselves feeling "connected to" or "a part of" something greater than ourselves.

This discovery process continues the theme explored in the last chapter. To have and give nurturing requires surrender—we must allow ourselves to trust others, and we must accept that we do have needs. Our Second Step, then, extends this basic premise. We move from the sense of "I have needs" and "There is purpose in all this" to a new place where we can acknowledge that both nurturing and sensuality are teaching us that we are connected to a larger life purpose—one in which we have a role. We may not understand that role, but we can begin to live it. We begin to trust that good things will come to us as part of our relationship with a Higher Power, and such trust brings comfort.

Thus, our senses may be regarded as the gateway to a spiritual life, with marveling at and wondering about creation coming first. Exploring sensuality leads to exploring the existence of a purpose or power greater than ourselves. If, however, we block our sensuality, we in turn block our spirituality.

Again, there's no magic switch for turning on our senses, just as none exists for nurturing. If we are not sensual in general, we will not suddenly be sensual when we are sexual. Healthy sexuality grows out of the way we live our lives—minute by minute, hour by hour, day by day. When we incorporate nurturing and sensuality into our day-to-day lives, they will naturally become part of our sexual lives.

Many of us greatly ignore much of the richness available to us through our senses—and to be sexual, we must first be capable of sensuality. And being open to sensuality requires being open to nurturing. If we can nurture ourselves, and allow others to nurture us as well, and if we can allow ourselves to be sensual, then we must also be able to accept and experience pleasure. Sexuality, sensuality, and spirituality are fundamentally linked. Healthy sexuality requires exploring one's spirituality.

Ultimately, therefore, we are on a spiritual journey—a

journey that begins at a very basic level with openness. When we at last open to the world of the senses, we become open to being nurtured. Nurturing requires trust and acceptance and dependence on another—trust that we'll be taken care of. And with openness and trust come the beginning recognition of greater connections, of synchronicity and serendipity. We realize there is more to our lives and more to the world than we ever imagined. We are part of—connected to—all that is around us.

Recognizing ourselves to be a part of the greater whole and *feeling* our interconnectedness form the fundamental basis of relationships. That recognition and feeling in turn sustain the kind of intimacy and respect and integrity that goes into the sexual transaction. Sensuality in its broadest sense, then, allows us to connect with our own feelings and those of others. Once we have made such a connection, it becomes increasingly difficult to be abusive, to exploit others, or to objectify them sexually.

It Takes Time to Be Sensual

Allowing ourselves to be sensual produces another unexpected phenomenon: Our sense of time is altered. If we're taking time to notice what's going on around us, then we can't be so caught up in society's driving pace—and that leaves time and freedom to play. I don't know how many couples have sat in my office and told me how they were once very attracted to each other, but now, after some years of marriage, the attraction is gone. It isn't until everything's fallen apart and they're in treatment that they ask what's happening. "Where did our romance go?" they wonder.

Part of what happened is that they let themselves become so busy that they no longer played. Romance has much to do with the fun of play and discovery. Think about how new couples act with one another. They spend a lot of time together, time doing "nothing" or playing or walking in parks or eating out or talking and talking or watching sunsets or listening to the rain in the trees—uninterrupted and playful *sensual* time together discovering each other and the world. They're not necessarily trying to accomplish something.

If we're so busy that we can't pay attention to ourselves and the world around us—to be sensual, in other words—we won't notice our partner, either. Couples need to have "windows" through which they notice animals, flowers, birds, a cool breeze—the world around them in all its beauty and richness. They need to play, and that requires the ability and willingness to trust and to let go.

Children are so good at play because they haven't become so busy yet; instead, they live in and give themselves over to the moment. They notice so much that we just take for granted or simply overlook as we busily charge through our lives.

I was reminded of this one day some years ago when I came to pick up my daughter Jennifer from school. I had just left work, and I was furious, though about what I can't even remember anymore. It's important to know that this was late March, and in Minnesota, that doesn't necessarily mean spring has arrived. That year, snow was still on the ground.

Jennifer was out on the playground, and when I saw her, I said, "Jennifer, it's time to go." She replied, "No Dad, I have something to show you first." I was in a bad mood anyway, and so I took this as defiance on her part and decided I had to insist on a limit.

"No, Jennifer, we have to leave now," I said demandingly. Well, this little child looked right up at me and said, with hand on hip, "Daaaaad, this is *impoorrrtant*." She then dragged me over to the wall of the school where the warmth of the sun had melted a little swath of ground. And there, in the middle of it, was a single green clover. My daughter had found the first green leaves in the state of Minnesota!

Fortunately, I had been able to shake myself away from whatever had angered me and let myself realize what an

141

astounding discovery she'd made. If I had kept "on track," however, and stuck to my goal of getting home ASAP, I would have missed this little miracle.

Imagine a group of kids playing tag or climbing trees. Do you think they're worrying about what they forgot to do the day before or what they have to do next week or tomorrow or even two hours from now? An absurd thought, isn't it! Kids know naturally how to live in the moment.

Pause for a moment now, and try to remember the times when you have felt most peaceful. Make a mental list of them.

When I ask patients to do this, I often hear such responses as "When I used to go fishing with my dad" or "When I was in the Grand Canyon" or "When I was canoeing." I find that very often these times of peace come when people are absorbed in and connected to nature. This sense of peace and connectedness is really a spiritual moment; and, while some of us find such moments in church, temple, or synagogue, it's not at all uncommon to find this feeling triggered by natural beauty or wonder.

If we have another person with us in such a moment, we can further anchor such moments in our memories. This connection in peace and calm, while moving and spiritual, is also basically playful and fun. Within this context, tremendous passion and intimacy are possible—and this core calmness and connection help create the trust needed to let go and play and be passionate with our partner.

And it all starts with a basic sensuality. We notice what is happening in our bodies and how our bodies respond to the world. Then we begin to notice and delight in and to assist our partner with his or her responses. We're experiencing and sharing this special moment with one another. All of this is needed to make the sexual experience healthy and fulfilling, but again, it can't happen with the snap of a finger. Nor will it occur the moment we decide to be sexual.

Healthy sex is in large part made up of play. It's not a driven rush to orgasm; instead, it's taking time to notice yourself and your partner. If you're not paying attention to the world in and around you, and you're not taking time to be sensual and playful in other parts of your life, you won't find playfulness in your sex life, either.

Cultural Bias against Pleasure and Sexuality

Cultivating a genuine delight in sensuality, playfulness, and pleasure runs contrary to a bias in Western culture dating back to Plato. Plato posited two worlds: an ideal one and the world in which we actually live. This idea is known as Platonic dualism, with the real world clearly inferior to the ideal world. The Apostle Paul, in turn, adapted this idea when he wrote of the kingdom of God, or heaven, toward which Jesus was leading humanity. Heaven, of course, was spiritual and perfect, contrary to a physical world filled with sin. The same idea was later immortalized in St. Augustine's *The City of God*.

Although Martin Luther had some profound disagreements with the Christianity of his time, he nevertheless accepted the Augustinian dualist view of the world. Being spiritual meant denying the body, which was basically lust-driven and evil. The needs and desires of the body, regardless of how pleasurable or natural, were to be spurned if one were to have any hope of redemption and happiness in the next life—to reach heaven, in other words.

Our cultural ambivalence about pleasure and sex has been carried forward through the centuries from Plato into Christianity via St. Paul and St. Augustine, and finally spreading into the various branches of Christianity after Martin Luther's reformation.

With such a long tradition of antisexual, antipleasure bias, it should not be surprising that to experience pleasure or provide another with pleasure—to be sensual—is also connected with shame for many people today. We try, unfortunately, to deny ourselves sensual feelings; yet the more we deny them, the stronger they become. Out of this situation grow binge-purge phenomena. Western culture has long been hedonistic and pleasure seeking, while at the same time believing such pleasure is bad and evil. We have a long history of being sex aversive, the result of which is that many people feel tremendous guilt and shame about sex.

I'm saying here that it's fine and good to allow ourselves to be nurtured, to be sensual, and to be sexual, and, more fundamentally, that we are basically good people who are redeemable.

A Modern-day Myth

This attitude of body avoidance, while having very old roots in our culture, is being reinforced by very modern forces too—the forces of technology. In one of our modern-day mythological tales, the *Star Wars* trilogy, Darth Vader, once a Jedi knight (striving for and defending all that is good and right), succumbed to the temptation of the Dark Side—the promise of immortality and power, the promise of godliness to be achieved mechanically. Vader became a consciousness kept alive by a machine—a human reaching for immortality through technology. By replacing his living, sensual body parts, however, Vader lost the essential limitation that helps humans keep a perspective on life. In this myth, George Lucas, the trilogy's creator and director, tells us that the great temptation in our time is to believe that our *technology* is our salvation—to believe that we can afford to ignore our bodies, our senses, and, in so doing, ignore our fundamental humanity.

The ancient Greeks introduced the concept of *hubris*—an arrogance about one's ability, a sense that one can become a god despite being human. Many Greek tragic heroes and heroines were good individuals striving with the best of intentions. Their downfall inevitably came, however, as the result of a fatal flaw: They denied their human limitations. In a similar vein, Ernest Becker argues persuasively in his 1974 Pulitzer-prize-winning book, *The Denial of Death*, that nearly all mental illness and addiction can be traced to issues of human limitation and our awareness and acceptance of it. And what is our ultimate limitation? The death of the body.

Living in a culture that promises ever-longer life through technological medicine makes it seductively easy to begin thinking we could be gods. This view sees the human body as nothing more than replaceable parts, with surgeons as the body mechanics. We strive to create modular bodies, and, as we do, we lose our sense of our limitations. This arrogance, as the Greeks taught so long ago, will lead to our downfall.

Technological disassociation from bodily limitations connects very closely to issues of sensuality. Philippe Aries, in his book *The Hour of Our Death*, points out that the rise of science and our ever-increasing technological competence have led us to become more and more "death negative."[1] In earlier times, people readily acknowledged their mortality. In many cultures both past and present, at the approach of death, an individual would call family and friends together and have the last talk and good-byes. In our culture today, many people find it enormously difficult to talk about death or to deal with someone close who's dying. Certainly we can talk easily and at length about those we don't know who die in accidents such as plane crashes, but if, for example, our next-door neighbor is dying of cancer, that's often a very different story. We don't know what to say or how to act.

Since the advent of the Industrial Revolution 150 years ago, Western culture has increasingly disengaged itself from the body. The emerging worldview, in which we see ourselves as unlimited and like unto a god, has taken us out of our bodies. In a sense, it is just a more modern edition of *The City of God* in which we increasingly ignore ourselves and our own nature.

We have become more body negative and death negative, and, without our being aware of it, our sexuality has become an inadvertent casualty. Historians note that the intensification of sexual repression started around the seventeenth and eighteenth centuries, when, in the West, we began to "fall in love" with machines and technology. The more we cut ourselves off from our senses, the less sexual we can be. Today, we deal poorly not only with death but also with sex. We've become sex negative as well.

The antidote for this situation, not just for the sexual anorexic but for all of us, is reconnecting and appreciating and caring for and listening to our bodies. By reconnecting with ourselves, we draw closer to our Source. And this Source is not only the fount of creativity and peace, but also of discernment, or a sense of knowing the truth. It is the knowing of what is right and what fits and what works *for oneself*. It is the ability to trust one's own judgment. This intuitive knowing is perhaps *the* most critical faculty we have, and it's so important for our sexual recovery. If we can't trust our own judgment, then we will act too cautiously—and that leads to overprotection of self and closing off to others and the world around us.

If, on the other hand, we have a good sense of discernment, we will know when to trust others, when a situation is right, and when it's safe to be open. We will have a *feeling* of correctness. And the fact is, we are most in touch with our inner self—our inner knowing—when we are most connected. This is absolutely critical for healthy sexuality. We simply can't give ourselves over to passion without a sense of knowing that the situation is safe and right.

KEY QUESTIONS

In workshops and in my counseling experience, the following questions are often asked when we talk about becoming more sensual.

Sex is never what I fantasize it to be—why am I always so disappointed?

For many people, a wide gap exists between sexual reality and sexual fantasy. This is primarily because their fantasies aren't anchored in their life experiences.

In studying the effectiveness of visualization for learning sports skills, researchers have looked at two basic techniques. In one, the athletes watch themselves going through the routine they are trying to perfect. In the other, the athletes imagine themselves actually doing the routine, and they try to include as many feelings and sensations and details about what they are working toward as they can.

Studies have found the second technique to be far more effective than the first. The more we can place ourselves in an imaginary sequence of events, the more effective the visualization in helping us learn. For example, if we want a better backhand in tennis, the most effective visualization would be one in which we are on the court, feeling the heat of the sun and the perspiration on our bodies, seeing and hearing the ball come off our opponent's racquet, watching it spin toward us, feeling our bodies as we move to the ball, feeling and hearing the impact of the ball off the racquet, and watching as it sails to exactly the spot we intended.

In other words, the most effective visualizations are anchored in reality and include as many feelings and sensations and details about what we are working toward as possible.

In sexual fantasies, people are disappointed when they imagine situations and partners that are simply out of the range of possibility. To avoid disappointment, we need to anchor our fantasies in our reality, and we need to make them as sensual as we can. (See the exercises at the end of this chapter.)

How do I become more sensual when I am so busy and involved? If I have no time for sex, how will I have time to be sensual?

The question is actually stated backwards. To find time for sex, we must first learn to slow down our lives, create windows for sensuality, and pay attention to and connect with our senses and feelings. Then, and only then, will we find a place for sex in our lives. If we don't have time to be sensual, we'll never have time for healthy sex, either.

ISSUES

When working on their sensuality, many sexual anorexics struggle with issues such as the following. Some of these issues have been explored at greater length in this or previous chapters; for those which have not, a brief discussion is included here. Read the issues carefully, noting the ones that apply to you. Then use those issues as discussion points with your partner and/or fair witnesses.

- Focusing on the present (as opposed to preoccupation about the past and worry about the future).
- Beginning self-awareness as a gateway to personal and spiritual growth.
- Confronting blocks around fear of touch or sound or visual fears.
- Learning to trust oneself and one's own reality.

Many of us have made promises to ourselves that we didn't keep. We weren't able to stay true to ourselves. Sometimes, of course, this happened because we experienced situations in which it was dangerous for us to be true to ourselves. Our goal now is to begin building trust—in both ourselves and in others. That begins by taking care of ourselves and by tuning in to what our senses tell us. We realize we are getting information that is important and useful, information that will ultimately bring us the ability to listen to our inner voice—and to act on what we hear. This is learning to have a sense of ourselves and to see the world as it is.

Sensuality

When we can pay attention to what our senses are telling us, we begin to connect to the larger world around us and to the world of nature. This is the gateway to personal and spiritual growth.

✿ Discovering that denial of reality is, in part, denial of the senses, and overcoming fear of body awareness.

We have already talked at some length about the loss of connection with our senses and factors involved in this condition. There is, however, an additional component to this problem. Some victims of abuse don't want to have body awareness. Why? Because with that awareness can come very painful memories. For these people, obliterating the senses was an important and useful coping mechanism at one time. Denying an awful reality made sense. Getting in touch again with feelings can be terribly frightening because of the horrible memories it might call up.

Given this, however, it's again important to remember what we explored in the previous chapter. We need to open ourselves to pain as a crucial part of the healing process.

Many in the counseling and medical professions have had a rather narrow approach to dealing with problems such as sexual anorexia. We've tried to "fix" people's sexuality as though it were nothing more difficult than putting a new computer component in the car.

Sexual anorexia and sexual addition, however, are *very* complex and interrelated. Five quick sessions with a counselor aren't enough. Not if we can't be nurtured. Not if we've shut down all our senses. If our fundamental, existential position in life is set to do things contrary to our being sexual, no number of new sexual techniques will overcome it. But when people follow the process outlined here, they find that they *can* change. The process works.

✿ Relying on obsession for reality.

This issue can be easily illustrated with a true story about a man I'll call "Scott." One evening, Scott was out cruising to pick up a woman when he pulled up next to a car at a stoplight. He and the woman driving the car exchanged glances. Scott thought she was flirting with him, so he followed her, his obsessive thinking shifting into ever-higher gears along with his car. He thought she was heading for a bar, and he imagined drinks, conversation, and, eventually, sex.

In the meantime, this woman pulled up and parked next to a large brick building. Scott, thinking they were at a bar, had one leg out of his car before he realized they were, in fact, in front of a police station! This poor woman was so frightened of Scott that she drove straight to the police, and Scott didn't even notice.

Scott had become disconnected from reality. This woman was frightened to death, and he thought she was coming on to him. For many addicts, obsession literally becomes reality.

🏶 Relying on others' perceptions of reality.
One of the ways that people become blocked in their sexuality is by relying on other people for their perceptions. This brings us back again to the importance of paying attention to our *own* senses. Learning to be sensual means learning to trust your *own* senses, your *own* perception of the world—*not* someone else's. Sexuality is, at its core, sensuality, and when we listen to ourselves, sensuality becomes another way to trust our own perceptions, our own reality—and sexuality becomes a way to be honest with ourselves, to be clear about our own truth.

TASKS

This chapter explores sensuality and its importance to healthy sexuality. It is through the senses—seeing, touching, smelling, hearing, tasting—that we come to know and enjoy the world. Our ability to work, to feel pleasure, to communicate with others, and to affect the world is directly related to our use of sensory energy. Everywhere, however, there is sad evidence that many of us have "lost our senses." The noise of dishwashers, air conditioners, power tools, and other appliances invades our space from every direction. We tax our sense of taste by eating and drinking foods that are too hot or too cold. The more our senses are overloaded, the more we withdraw from sensory stimulation.

We can, however, reclaim our senses quite easily. We need only take a little time and effort to pay attention to them—and that is exactly what the following exercises are designed to do—expand your ability to be sensual.

SENSORY EXERCISES[2]

The following exxercises are based on material from Bernard Gunther's *Sense Relaxation*.[2] You may want to do these exercises with your partner—one of you can read the directions while the other does the exercise. Then, switch roles.

Have fun! Discover! Remember!

WASHING YOUR HANDS AND ARMS

Standing before a bathroom sink, adjust the water to a pleasant lukewarm temperature. Close your eyes and slowly lather your hands with soap. Take your time. The main idea is to be fully conscious of the process and of the sensations experienced. Move the lather up and around both arms all the way to the elbow. Feel the skin against skin contact, the lubrication of the soap, the temperature of the lather. Hear the water rushing, and smell the fragrance of the soap. Rinse both hands and arms and feel the cooling of your skin in the air. Slowly lather your arms and hands and rinse again, again noting all the details of the experience. Dry your hands and feel the texture and friction of the towel against hands, against arms.

Paying Close Attention

Close your eyes. Tune in to the sounds of the room. Listen to and feel your breathing, the heave of your chest, the drop of your diaphragm, the distinct sounds of inhalation and exhalation. Feel the air temperature on your face and hands. Feel the clothing draped on your body, and become aware of yourself as inside the clothes, as inhabiting them. Note and feel the contact points between clothing and skin. Become aware of the sensation of your feet pressing on the floor, and of your arms and hands resting on your legs or the arms of a chair.

Stretching

Lie flat on your back on the floor with eyes closed. Feel your body against the floor, noting the contact points between floor and body. Without strain, begin stretching each part of your body, starting at the toes and feet and moving upward—ankles, calves, knees, thighs, hips, buttocks, stomach, chest, shoulders, arms, wrists, fingers, neck, face, and scalp—experiencing each sensation in turn. Where is there pain or discomfort? Where are there particularly pleasurable sensations?

Using Your Subordinate Hand

For at least thirty minutes, try using your subordinate hand—the left if your are right-handed, the right if you are left-handed—as you go about your daily business. Try drinking from a cup, zipping zippers, opening doors, turning pages with the opposite hand you would normally use to do these things. Be aware of the sensations and your feelings about the effort—your frustrations, your patience (or lack thereof), perhaps the humor of the experience. When your stop the experiment, note how you feel about yourself.

Sensuality

PEELING AN ORANGE

Place an orange in the palm of your hand and examine it visually. Note the shape, texture, color, unique markings, or anomalies. Smell the skin of the orange. Close your eyes and roll the orange in your hands and up and down your forearms, noting its texture and firmness. Smack the orange with one hand, noting the sound it makes. Roll it across your face and shoulders and neck.

Slowly and gently break the skin of the orange and begin to remove the peel. Smell the odors, see and feel the juice on your skin, watch the skin as you tear it away in pieces, revealing the inner flesh of the fruit. Break the orange in half and separate a section from one of the halves. Do this as slowly as possible, feeling the flesh of the orange gradually give way. Close your eyes and place the section in your mouth, rolling it around with your tongue, feeling it against your cheeks, biting into it and feeling the juice flow out onto your tongue, tasting the pungent citrus flavor. Repeat this process with each section of the orange.

DINING IN SILENCE

With one other person or a group of people, eat an entire meal without speaking. Eat slowly. Closely observe the food and the company. Note the various smells and tastes and colors and arrangements and tactile sensations, the movement of your hands and arms and lips and jaw and tongue. Eat for a time while maintaining eye contact with your company. Eat for a time while your eyes are closed.

BARRIERS TO SENSUALITY

What rules do you live by, in general, that prevent you from being sensual when you're trying to be sexual? Write them in your journal.

A Sensual Fantasy

Imagination and the senses are inextricably linked. In this exercise, write a sensual fantasy. Make it as complete as you can by including information from all your senses. You might, for example, imagine yourself in a quiet park, leaning against a tree. What would you see? Hear? Smell? Be aware of your sense of touch and taste (perhaps you're eating an ice-cream cone). Write your imagined experience in your journal.

A Sexual Fantasy

✐ In this exercise, take what you practiced and learned in the previous exercise and write a sensual *sexual* fantasy. Again include information from all the senses as much as you are able. Write your imagined experience in your journal.

Sharing Fantasies

Share what you have written in the previous two exercises with your partner. Pay particular attention to the differences between the two imagined experiences.

Erotic Observations

Over the course of a week, pay attention to the things about your partner that you find erotic. Don't limit yourself to the blatantly sexual, however. Perhaps you find erotic the curve of an arm, the way muscles flex during some task, the way a particular shirt hangs off a shoulder, his or her hair, a particular look, and so on. Write these things down as you notice them.

At the week's end, share what you've noticed with each other.

PLANNING

For the next week or two, decide on specific ways you can incorporate more sensuality into your life.

- What specific ways can you allow yourself to be sensual?
- How will you know that you are being sensual?

Share this plan with your group, therapist, or sponsor (your "fair witnesses") to get their input and suggestions too.

IN YOUR JOURNAL

Start each morning by writing your "daily pages." In addition, since this chapter focuses on sensuality, create a momentary sensual inventory. Notice what's going on with your body—including any sensual sexual feelings. Write down exactly what you are feeling each morning.

The famous human sexuality research team of Masters and Johnson stated that one must learn to talk about sex before, during, and after sex. Paying attention to, writing about, and then sharing these intimate feelings with your partner is a way to begin talking about your sexual experiences. By acknowledging these feelings to yourself and to another, you begin to make your sexuality explicit—and this eventually will pay wonderful dividends.

A CLOSING EXERCISE

The closing exercise asks you and your partner to evaluate yourselves and one another. Remember, this exercise offers a wonderful opportunity for you to discover your strengths and weaknesses, as well as a chance for you and your partner to compare your perceptions of yourselves and one another.

In addition to filling out the rating scales, it will be helpful to do the following:

- Once you have filled out your scales, share the results with your fair witnesses.
- After your partner has finished, talk about your partner's perceptions too. They may differ from yours and/or those of your fair witnesses.

- If significant discrepancies exist, note them and then return to your fair witnesses to look into them more carefully.

As you work on these scales, try not to become defensive if the perceptions your partner or your fair witnesses have of you differ from your own perceptions of yourself. Let these differences—and the reasons for them—be a source of information for all of you.

If you are not currently in a relationship, ask one of your fair witnesses (therapist, sponsor, anorexia group member, Twelve Step support group member, or RCA group member, for example) to work through the scales with you.

Part 1: Focus on You

Consider sensuality as it applies to you. How open are you to your senses? Do you pay attention to what your senses tell you? How much work do you need on sensuality to feel comfortable with your skills?

Circle your rating on the scale below. (1 = low skills, need much work; 10 = high skills, need no further work.)

Next, ask your partner to think about your sensuality. On the same scale below, have your partner use a square to rate you.

1	2	3	4	5	6	7	8	9	10

Part 2: Focus on Your Partner

On this second scale, ask your partner to consider his or her own sensuality. How much does your partner pay attention to what his or her senses are saying? How much work does your partner need to feel comfortable with his or her sensuality?

Have your partner use a circle to rate himself or herself.

Next, you rate your partner's skills and ability in this area. Use a square to do so.

1	2	3	4	5	6	7	8	9	10

Sensuality

Nurturing—
We learn to trust and to open our lives to experience.

Sensuality—
Through our senses, we interact with the world around us
and become connected to it.

SELF-IMAGE

The dark night gave me a pair of dark eyes.
I am using them to seek the light.

—Gu Cheng

WHEN WE LOOK at self-image, the basic theme of chapters 6 and 7 again plays the crucial role. Our sexuality cannot be separated from the rest of our being. Without the ability to nurture and be sensual, our sexual lives will disappoint us. Likewise, for sex to feel good, we have to feel deserving and attractive and positive about ourselves. If our overall self-image is poor, it will necessarily affect the sexual part of our lives. Problems with self-image, in fact, become more difficult and complex when sexuality comes into play. Our self-image is like a lens through which we view our lives. Nothing goes as well—or as well as it might—if we are not feeling good about ourselves.

The image we as adults have about our sexuality forms, like so much of our personality, during childhood. Our early sexual experiences create a template of what we find attractive and arousing, and out of these experiences emerge a "story line" about what is connected with our sexual arousal.

Most people never pay any attention to their story line, never realize, in fact, that they even have one. It just seems to work for them. Others, however, feel embarrassed or ashamed over what they find arousing, as the following stories of Alicia and Bob show, and thus live with a damaged sexual self-image. As a young woman, Alicia discovered that the only way that she could masturbate and achieve orgasm was by using a blanket in a tightly constricted manner. This can be, of course, more than a little awkward and cumbersome, not to mention that it's rather difficult to involve a partner. When she wants to be sexual with someone, Alicia feels great embarrassment about this and consequently has long believed that something is wrong with her because she's not "normal."

Bob grew up in a poor rural area, and his home had no indoor toilets. At some point, Bob began to hide behind the family's outhouse to listen and watch while the women in the family were urinating. As he grew a little older, urination became associated with his sexual arousal—and this was profoundly shameful to him. He was aware enough to know that in this culture, most people do not find urination erotic, and so he concluded that he was, in fact, a bad and perverted person—a sexual self-image he carried well into his adult life.

All of us develop a sexual self-image that increasingly comes into focus as we grow into adults, and all of us struggle somewhat with our sexual self-image because we live in a culture that is virtually unable to teach its children about sex. In many, many families, talk about sexuality is basically off-limits, thus children never have the opportunity to discuss their sexual feelings or inclinations with their parents. Kids want to know whether or not what they feel is normal because feeling sexual is completely new to them. They simply aren't at all sure of themselves. But because they receive little, if any, feedback or support from parents, teachers, or other adults, and because they're usually unwilling to ask friends for fear of ridicule, their sexual feelings remain hidden and secret. Imagine the struggle homosexuals and bisexuals must endure to achieve a positive sexual self-image.

When we perceive our sexuality to be outside the norm—or

for whatever reason "weird"—damage to our sexual self-image occurs, which, in turn, magnifies feelings of defectiveness in our overall self-image. From these essential conclusions about our sexual selves can emerge a belief, based in shame and secrecy, that no one who really knew us would ever want to be with us sexually.

This difficult situation can be further exacerbated when we grow up in an environment of abuse or neglect. In such cases, we come to the conclusion that we're basically bad or unworthy people whom others wouldn't like at all if they really knew us. We feel that although sex is a very important need, no one would want to be sexual with us because they wouldn't like us as people. Add to this mix sexual preferences or arousal scenarios that we think are strange, and the result is a tight internal logic that bars us from wanting to be open and vulnerable.

Children who have been sexually abused will have, of course, varied reactions to those experiences. One conclusion they draw is that the only way they can be liked by others is to be sexual with them. Although at an intuitive level such children know that abuse is wrong and that they shouldn't have to participate, they nevertheless come away from these experiences with the sense that *they* somehow acted wrongly. The result is increasingly damaged self-esteem and ever-greater feelings of helplessness.

By the time one is an adult, these experiences and feelings about self can come together to produce an internal logic that has very destructive outcomes. Alicia's childhood experiences of sexual abuse led her to believe as an adult that the only way she could please men was to be sexual with them. But Alicia doesn't *feel* sexual, so instead she fakes it. Alicia wants to have men with her, but to have a man in her life, she realizes, has required her to be essentially dishonest. She feels, too, that any man who's in her life under such terms must fundamentally be living a charade—she's not worth liking so he must be only pretending to like her.

Combine these feelings with an arousal story line that is deeply embarrassing to her, and Alicia experiences her intimate relationships as a house of cards just waiting to fall. She's never truly herself, and consequently she repeatedly finds herself in repulsive and destructive relationships. It's a cycle that never gives Alicia what she really wants while further damaging her self-image every time it repeats. As you can see, early sexual history can be of great significance because of the key conclusions it leads us to make about ourselves and about our sexuality.

What Is "Attractive"?

The other very important conclusion that emerges from our early childhood experiences is what it means to be an attractive man and an attractive woman—and these conclusions are affected by one's gender and sexual orientation. A woman, for example, will eventually decide what would make her, as a woman, attractive to men, what kind of men she would be attracted to, and what kind of men would be attracted to the woman she is—or would like to be. These assumptions all play a part in her sexuality. Being gay or lesbian further complicates this process. These gender and gender-orientation issues profoundly affect how we feel in general about ourselves and how we feel in particular about our sexual selves.

A story from my own life illustrates both how such assumptions play out in our lives as well as how unaware of them we can be. If you're old enough, you might remember an ad for bodybuilding that regularly ran on the back pages of comic books. The title read: *Are you a 97-pound weakling?* The ad showed in cartoon form a skinny fellow at the beach with his pretty girlfriend. Soon a big, muscular guy walks over, kicks sand in the weakling's face, and says he wants the girl. The weakling, of course, is no match for Mr. Muscles, who walks away with the poor guy's girl. He sits dejectedly, wishing he, too, were big and strong. Enter Charles Atlas, a bodybuilder who gives the pitch about how, if the weakling buys and uses Atlas's special work-out machine, he will never again lose his girl.

When I was eleven years old and reading those comic books, I weighed exactly ninety-seven pounds. I knew, absolutely *knew,* that those ads were meant for me. So I honest-to-God sent away for this machine. I wanted a body like that guy. I thought, as did many men, that what really attracted women were big arms. A muscular body. I just assumed that this was what women wanted. Ads like this were part of the way I came to this conclusion, and I acted on this belief. I tried to match my self-image with what I thought women wanted.

Now we know, of course, that many women are actually *repelled* by bodybuilder-type bodies. The physical attributes most women, in fact, say they pay attention to (leaving emotional concerns aside for the moment!) are eyes, thinness, and butts. Women are attracted to thin men with nice eyes and cute butts. When I tell this story to audiences, this always brings squeals from the women. They recognize the truth here! Yet how many men still think women want Charles Atlas—and try to measure themselves against that standard? This is yet-another classic example of learning, acting on, and having one's self-image negatively affected by misinformation and misconceptions about sexuality.

Women, of course, have similar experiences. A recent television news show aired a segment on a Cindy Crawford cover shot for a national magazine. Despite Crawford's having a body that fits our culture's ideal for women, the magazine nevertheless digitized the photo and used its computers to make her legs and arms thinner, remove shadows and wrinkles, enhance skin tones, and otherwise alter her body—changes impossible to discern in the finished photo. Ultimately, this was no longer a photo of a human being. It was a computer-enhanced image that does not exist in the real world—a truly unachievable ideal. Yet women see such photos and think that this is what men want. They work very hard to achieve not only an impossible ideal, but also one in which many men have little interest.

In forming our sexual self-image, many of us—men and women alike—put ourselves up against unrealistic and nearly mythological ideals of what's attractive, and when we inevitably fall short of the ideal, our conclusions about our sexuality are needlessly affected for the worse.

Our sexuality and sexual self-image are also affected by another process that we avoid thinking about or discussing. Aging, if you're older than twenty-five or thirty, you've certainly noticed that certain parts of your body can settle into places on your frame other than where you've been accustomed to finding them previously! As we get older, our bodies shift and change; they no longer look like they did when we were eighteen. These physical changes require a shift in how we continue to feed our sexual self-image. Learning to see and accept the stretch marks and thinning, graying hair, for example, as changes you've earned by living will help make them feel positive. We can cherish these changes as "badges" of a sort that are physical manifestations of what we've lived through.

I have some balding spots on my head, for example, which my kids teased me about when they were younger. They'd often say, "Dad, you're growing through your hair." After a while, I became somewhat sensitive about this. But then I realized that as a parent (and a single parent, at that), there were too many times during the day when I'd hit myself on the head and say, "You did WHAT!?!?" So I began telling the kids that I was actually wearing out the hair there! I earned those bald spots. By getting to this point, I was able to normalize the situation for myself; I came to see my bald spots as a kind of badge of courage—courage to live in the world. When our sexuality is based on relationship and love, rather than just physical looks, our sexual self-image is far more realistic—and we will not find our sex lives diminished by the inevitable physical changes.

As adults, we have, over the years, accumulated a relationship history that we bring to the present. If past sexual relationships were very passionate, yet ended in pain for us, it's possible for us to begin connecting passion with rejection. We then fear new relationships. Similarly, people who have abandoned relationships, who have acted unfaithfully, or who have feared a past lover (or lovers) may see themselves as untrustworthy—and rightfully so, since they *have* been. And since they have had little success at sustaining and maintaining a relationship, they have little confidence in their ability to succeed in future relationships.

Regardless of why we feel diminished, this feeling can affect our sense of self—and our sense of how attractive we are to a potential partner. Without a good sense of self, we can find ourselves increasingly isolated and caught in a self-fulfilling prophecy. When we don't feel genuinely attractive, others can conclude that something is wrong with us—and consequently aren't attracted to us. What may start out as a good relationship will self-destruct because of our expectation that it can't work; after all, none of our past relationships have worked. We learn to distrust any kind of sexual meeting because we've "been down that road before," and it's proven too often to have a bad end. Ultimately, we hold ourselves at a distance from everyone, further diminishing the possibility of relationship.

There Is a Way Out

One of the measures we can take to break this cycle is to surround ourselves with good people whom we trust and who are important to us. Though we are ultimately striving to reach a point where we can affirm our self-esteem from within, we can begin building it with the help of others. Receiving care from others reinforces the idea that we *do* deserve a better life, that we are good, worthwhile people. This is the lesson supportive families teach their children when they provide an environment that includes unconditional love and acceptance. Children thus learn that despite their mistakes, they will be loved and cared for—and that's how good self-esteem develops and flourishes.

Those who don't get unconditional love from their families need to find it someplace else, and one of the ways this can take place is through Twelve Step programs, sponsors, therapists—and our fair witnesses. We can finally involve ourselves with people who will love and support us, despite our mistakes—people who will be here for us when we need them and help and affirm us on this path. In such an environment, our self-esteem can't help but grow.

As our self-esteem grows and we begin to feel better about ourselves, it's not unusual to find that we begin to pay more attention to our physical health and appearance. At this point, exercise can play an important role in further healing.

Regular exercise positively affects our bodies. We have more energy and feel a greater sense of well-being. Taking better care of ourselves physically can also significantly affect our sex lives, including our ability to achieve orgasm.

I know it's difficult to work exercise into the day. There are certainly some nights when I'm so tired that my view of exercise is to sit in a nice hot tub for a while, and then pull the plug and fight the current! People who don't feel very good about themselves don't feel much like putting energy into taking care of themselves, nor do they take much pride in how they look or appear. The presentation of self just doesn't matter if you don't feel very good about yourself to begin with.

But once you begin feeling better about yourself, you'll find you have the energy to take better care of yourself in many ways—and the exercises at the end of this chapter will help you begin this process. You'll find that the vicious cycle of poor self-image/poor body image/low energy can be turned on its head. As we exercise, for example, we soon feel and look better physically, and consequently begin to feel better about ourselves in general. Feeling better about ourselves, we also find that we have more energy to exercise. But we have to start somewhere.

The Importance of Others

As we talk about developing a more positive self-image, I can't help but remember my days as a graduate student at Brown University many years ago. It was common for many of the grad students to gather in the student union every morning for coffee and camaraderie. I remember getting my coffee and sitting down on the periphery of the group. I didn't drink my coffee, though, because I was so nervous about being there—my self-esteem then was practically nonexistent—that my hands would be shaking and I knew I would spill the coffee if I tried to drink it. This was a small incident, but looking back, it's clear now just how poor my self-image was. It's very gratifying to me that, some years later, after a lot of hard work, I can hold a cup a coffee and stand in front of audiences numbering sometimes in the thousands to speak. At long last, I have learned to really like being with myself.

As our self-image improves, we experience what the famous Catholic theologian Henri Nouwen describes in his book *Reaching Out* as the conversion of loneliness to solitude. This is the ability to be with one's self and not be afraid of the experience. It's the ability to develop a sense of trust in who you are.

We begin developing this ability by first allowing other people to care for us and affirm us. Next, by concentrating on our senses, we begin to trust *our* ability to know the outside world, thus fostering a wonderful sensual passion. We next find ourselves altering some of our fundamental conclusions about our lives. We realize that we are indeed worthwhile—and worth being with. From this evolves a better and better sense of who we are. To move further in our recovery, it *is* necessary to know what we are about.

Let me again illustrate these ideas with a personal experience. After an appearance on a national television program, I was feeling highly critical of myself. My wife encouraged me to call a good friend—an older woman who lived near my home in Minnesota. I called Ann and, after our customary greetings and chitchat, we started talking about the show. She'd seen it, too, and had some of the same perceptions I did as far as the commentators not representing the topic and structuring the show in the way I'd anticipated.

At some point, however, Ann suddenly said, "But you know, I started thinking about how funny my toes are."

"Ann," I said. "*What* are you talking about?"

But she continued, "I've been thinking about how strange and weird toes are, but that if you start saying positive things to yourself each day about them, if you look at them in a different light, toes are really fun. Think about it, Pat! Each toe has a different job." And then Ann went on to describe the jobs toes have.

Finally, she said, "And then I step back and I look at the fact that the woodpecker at my feeder has this lovely red crest, and then I look at the morning sun on the poinsettia that you gave me for Christmas, and I feel *really* good about life."

Well, by now I found myself just laughing and thinking that, of course, *these* are the things that really count, and all the things I was upset over just aren't quite so important.

This story perfectly illustrates the connections we've been talking about. I had temporarily lost track of who I am because of my feelings of betrayal and public vulnerability. My being sensual—paying attention to what's around me and to the messages the world gives me—together with the help of a good and trusting friend, enabled me to return to my center and see what really matters, to recover my sense of who I really am as a person.

We're now talking about enjoying the experience of being you! Can you see how all of this fits together? If we can get to the place where we can see our sexuality—see how our bodies work and notice our responses—we will be more available to ourselves and, consequently, we will be more available to others. We'll find we have greater confidence in our ability to let others be close to us and to be close to others. Then, when someone is attracted to us, we won't be so surprised. As adults who are confident and who care for ourselves, we'll be able to say, "Of course, it's not a surprise that someone would find me attractive. I am a good, kind person who has something to offer." And we'll be better able to judge whether or not that person is appropriate for us.

Now we are living, not in a place of rejection and abandonment, but one in which we have a profound acceptance of ourselves. When we reach this level of acceptance, other people will see us as that person. They will respond not to an image we're projecting, but to the beautiful and worthwhile person we really are.

The Role of Trust of Self

One of the keys to a healthy sexual relationship is trust. In such a relationship, we don't try to be what someone else wants. The person we project is who we are. Such trust changes the fundamental dynamic of the relationship; it is characterized by authenticity and acceptance.

At this point, it's important to begin paying attention to how our feelings of desire make us feel about ourselves. Does what we desire make us feel bad about ourselves? When we ask such questions, we are led to reflect on a range of issues—our family lives, our upbringing, the messages we received from those with whom we lived while growing up, our early sexual experiences. All these messages and experiences have come together over the years—and we bring them to every relationship and sexual encounter we have. Our task here is to really look at ourselves.

From a Twelve Step perspective, this is the Third Step—we are trying to reach a point in our lives where we can accept ourselves as we are, and we can trust others. This is the point where change can really begin. We have to first know and accept who we are *now*. Clinical literature overwhelmingly shows that what we live through we carry with us and bring to our current reality. We become the person we believe ourselves to be—and this is why affirmations can be such a powerful tool for change. Changing our attitudes about life, ourselves, and the way we live is very difficult without the experience of seeing others who've successfully changed their lives and are living better and more happily because of it.

These first three Steps we take in this and the previous two chapters are closely interrelated. We awaken and look around to see the marvelous world that's around us. We begin to understand that a Higher Power exists and lives in us. We see and accept ourselves for who we are, and we allow nurturing into our lives. We decide to try to change ourselves, and we trust that, with the help of others, we can do so. We trust that if we "act as if" we are the person we want to be, we will be that person because reality will respond to the practice of that possibility.

KEY QUESTIONS

In workshops and in my counseling experience, the following questions are often asked in reference to self-image.

How do I affirm myself sexually when it's the other person's approval I seem to need?
The core point of this chapter speaks precisely to this question. We have lived far too long paying attention to the expectations of others and believing that "these are not *our* problems." Too often we expect others to be responsible for our sexual happiness, when instead we need to examine what we are doing and thinking. *We* are responsible for our sexual happiness. It starts with us, with our past experiences, our self-image, our expectations. Do we like

what we see and how we feel? As we have seen, at one level our sexual happiness and our sexual relationships have very little to do with other people. We need to start at that level.

I have felt sexually inadequate since childhood. How can that change now?

Change begins with believing that change is possible. I no longer sit quietly with a quivering hand spilling coffee. I've learned that I can trust myself and be successful, that people will appreciate who I am. It is possible to change. It may be hard to believe this, and it certainly doesn't happen overnight. We need to put in time and effort—and believe we can succeed.

ISSUES

Many sexual anorexics struggle with the following issues in reference to self-image. These issues have been explored at length in this or previous chapters. Read them carefully, noting the ones that apply to you. Then use those issues as discussion points with your partner and/or fair witnesses.

❀ Feeling ashamed of one's body image.

❀ Having performance fears.

❀ Fearing intimacy because of hurt and resentment about past experiences.

❀ Feeling untrustworthy because of past betrayals and infidelities.

❀ Distrusting others' attractions to oneself because of a poor self-image.

❋ Confronting negative "programming" from family and friends about one's sexuality and appearance.

❋ Learning to affirm oneself versus relying on feelings of inadequacy.

❋ Overcoming personal shame, supercharged expectations, and unrealistic notions about one's sexual self.

TASKS

One way you can begin to understand some of the issues we are looking at is to closely examine how you developed your attitudes about your sexual self and your story line. It's important to better understand how that map or template was established. In the following exercise, your task is to try to remember the messages you received about sex in general and your sexuality in particular as you were growing up.

Your Story Line

This exercise will help you identify key events or factors in your sexual history. Answer the questions by giving the approximate age and the specific event that was part of your sexual development. Write your answers in your journal.

1. What were your key childhood sexual experiences up to age ten (strong memories, traumatic events, events that evoke strong feelings, and child abuse by parents or other adults)?

2. What were your key adolescent sexual experiences up to age eighteen (sexual experimentation, masturbation, onset of menstruation, sexual abuse by family members or other adults, fantasy life, other)?

3. What were your key young adult sexual experiences up to

age twenty-five (dating, same-sex relationships, marriage, divorce, other)?

4. What were your key adult sexual experiences up to the present (include current sexual patterns)?

5. What impact might any or all of the following have had on your sexual development? Don't worry about "knowing" the "right" answer. Try to imagine what the possibilities may be. You can go back to your answers later and pick out those that make the most sense to you.

- How have family attitudes about sex affected your sexual development?

- How has religion affected your sexual development?

- How has your ethnic or cultural heritage affected your sexual development?

- How has your work or career affected your sexual development?

PLANNING

Others now in your life—your sponsor, fair witnesses, those in a support group—can help you "deprogram" yourself. They can help you transform your negative self-image to a positive self-image. For example, these people can assist you in writing affirmations about yourself. Decide on one or more ways you can work to strengthen your self-image. For the next month or two, strive to carry out your plans. Whenever possible, ask your support group, sponsor, or fair witnesses to help you. Here are some examples of concrete ways to build self-esteem.

- Accept unquestioningly any compliments others give you.

- Develop a visualization in which you care for yourself as you deserve to be cared for.

- Develop one or more affirmations to improve your self-image. Here are two examples:
  I am a person who feels good about who I am and how I look.
  When people make comments about how nice I look, or that I'm attractive, I will pay attention and not dismiss them.

- Go to your fair witnesses and ask them to give you accurate and honest feedback about yourself. You might ask, for example, about ways you are attractive.

- Ask your support group to let you know when they see you looking nice.

- If you are with a spouse or partner, set aside time to give each other examples of what attracts you to one another.

IN YOUR JOURNAL

Begin each morning by writing your "daily pages." Since this chapter focuses on self-image, create a momentary self-image inventory—a look at how you see yourself, how you feel about yourself, what you like or dislike about yourself at the moment you are writing. Include your feelings about your sexual self-image and sexual history.

A CLOSING EXERCISE

The closing exercise asks you and your partner to evaluate yourselves and one another. Remember, this exercise offers a wonderful opportunity for you to discover your strengths and weaknesses, as well as a chance for you and your partner to compare your perceptions of yourselves and one another.

In addition to filling out the rating scales, it will be helpful to do the following:

- Once you have filled out your scales, share the results with your fair witnesses.
- After your partner has finished, talk about your partner's perceptions too. They may differ from yours and/or those of your fair witnesses.
- If significant discrepancies exist, note them and then return to your fair witnesses to look into them more carefully.

As you work on these scales, try not to become defensive if the perceptions your partner or your fair witnesses have of you differ from your own perceptions of yourself. Let these differences—and the reasons for them—be a source of information for all of you.

If you are not currently in a relationship, ask one of your fair witnesses (therapist, sponsor, anorexia group member, Twelve Step support group member, or RCA group member, for example) to work through the scales with you.

Part 1: Focus on You

Consider your self-image. What do you think of yourself as a person? How do your see yourself? Is this similar to how others see you or quite different? How much work do you need on your self-image?

Using a circle, rate yourself on the scale below. (1 = low skills, need much work; 10 = high skills, need no further work.)

Next, ask your partner to rate how you think of yourself. Have your partner use a square to rate you.

1   2   3   4   5   6   7   8   9   10

Part 2: Focus on Your Partner

On this second scale, ask your partner to consider his or her own self-image. What does your partner think of himself or herself as a person? How does your partner see himself or herself? Is this similar to the view others have of your partner or quite different? How much work does your partner need on self-image?

Have your partner use a circle to rate himself or herself.

Next, you rate your partner on self-image. Use a square to do so.

I	2	3	4	5	6	7	8	9	10

Nurturing—
We learn to trust and to open our lives to experience.

Sensuality—
Through our senses, we interact with the world around us and become connected to it.

Self-Image—
We learn that we are good and lovable.

SELF-DEFINITION

Whatever the cost in personal relationships, we discover that our highest responsibility, finally, unavoidably, is the stewardship of our potential—being all that we can be. We betray this trust at the peril of our mental and physical health.

—Theodore Roszak

THE DEVELOPMENT OF SELF-DEFINITION begins very early in our lives. In *Identity and the Life Cycle*, psychologist and writer Erik Erikson showed years ago that infants have *already* made a decision by six months of age as to whether they can trust their caregivers and whether they're going to be taken care of.[1] Even at such a young age, our sense of self is already forming. As we grow in awareness, our first realization is of our senses and the information about our world that our senses bring us. We learn to trust and to open our lives to experience. We continue to explore the world, and through our senses, we interact with the world around us and become connected to it. Eventually, we find ourselves able to look at our place in that world. We also begin forming conclusions about who we are, thus developing our self-image. We learn that we are good and lovable. We develop a relationship with the self and come to trust ourselves. We see ourselves as trustworthy. And once we develop this foundational level of self-acceptance, we begin to define who we are as a person, to take a kind of inventory of what we—and life—are all about.

The early formation of self-definition is crucial to the issues we are examining because it's during these first four to five childhood years that so many sexual issues begin to assert themselves. What feels good and what does not, our preferences, our values all begin to come into play in our lives.

Many people who are struggling with sexual anorexia have had problematic life histories. They were sexual, for example, against their own wishes, or, conversely, they avoided sex when they were interested. They made promises to themselves to take certain actions, yet didn't follow through on them. As a result of such experiences, they lost their trust in themselves over time, and now no longer believe that what they say they're going to do will happen. At a basic level, then, they develop a distrust in their ability to operate in their own best interest. And one of the ways to deal with this belief is to not do anything—to totally shut down. This is exactly the anorexic or deprivation solution.

Boundaries and Their Development

The way an individual establishes and maintains personal boundaries reveals much about her or his sense of self-definition. Boundaries are incredibly significant in building relationships between people. At the most basic level, for a relationship to exist, two people need to be relating with one another. Two defined, separate selves. Without defined and clear boundaries, the needs, desires, problems, goals—all that make up a relationship—flow together in unhealthy ways. An old joke about a couple who had lived together for sixty years illustrates this problem: While out sightseeing during a vacation, the wife turns to her husband and says, "Honey, put on your coat, I'm cold."

Without self-definition, we have neither boundaries nor clear differentiation of who we are as individuals. When we lose that differentiation, we also lose the fundamental risks of intimacy that keep the vitality of relationships alive, as we shall see later.

The ability to define oneself is a prerequisite for the ability to set boundaries—to regulate how we will interact with another person, how close to another we'll allow ourselves to be, what's acceptable and what we absolutely will not tolerate. Self-definition also includes the ability and strength—the requisite self-respect—to say no when a boundary is breached: to tell others that when we say something, we mean it. Our boundaries are clear.

If loss of trust in one's self has occurred, holding boundaries can be difficult, and that creates even more distrust of self. Cari, for example, was a sexual abuse victim who often felt pressure from her partner to be sexual. She told him that being sexual with him was sometimes very difficult because she was now dealing with painful feelings from her past, and at such times she just needed to be with herself. Being sexual was more than she could handle at times. Her partner, however, often ignored her wishes, and Cari caved in to his demands. A fundamental violation of self-trust occurred when Cari let her partner continue to be sexual with her. She was unable to enforce the boundaries she'd set for herself. What's more, the result further confirmed Cari's distrust in her ability to take care of herself.

Distrust of self can cause an additional problem in our sexual relationships—it blocks our ability to experience passion. If we don't trust our ability to protect ourselves, we can't give ourselves over to our passion because we won't be certain of the outcome. When we ask ourselves, "Will I be safe?" the answer will be, "Maybe not." Passion is simply too frightening in such situations because we don't have a relationship with ourselves. To truly let go, we must be confident, at a very basic level, that we'll be safe.

The cornerstone of healthy sexuality is a relationship with

ourselves that works. When we have trouble with sex, the problem seldom lies in our partner or our circumstances or even our life histories, but rather with a significant distrust of ourselves.

Setting boundaries requires that we know both what we want and what we don't want. Buddhism describes this idea by saying that if you are going to say no, you must know what yes is. We *must* have a sense of where we are going in life. We need to have a vision of what we want to do—*and* we must note clearly what we do not want to do. Only then can we set our boundaries and direction in life.

Self-Definition: Looking at the Dark Side

Self-definition begins with nurturing, through which we acknowledge that we're worthy of care. Sensuality opens us up to receiving this care. A good self-image lets us see the positive value in all of these experiences. Self-definition enables us to take a stand about ourselves as persons.

As described by psychologist Carl Jung, the process of self-definition begins with looking at our dark side. Most of us prefer not to think of ourselves as having a "dark side," but we do. Each of us has, over the course of our lives, taken actions about which we'd rather not have the rest of the world know. All of us have done this.

Be assured that denial of the dark or shadow side is not unusual. On the contrary, it's common among people seeking treatment, and particularly so among addicts and anorexics who have large dark sides that they literally deny to both themselves and everybody around them.

To make this idea more clear, imagine a balloon filled with such feelings as resentment, jealousy, fear, anger, shame, loneliness, and pain. To deal with these feelings, addicts, codependents, and abuse survivors often build a false ego around their "balloon," and it's that false self that they present to the world.

When a therapist, treatment group member, or other person

calls them on their deceit, the reaction is very predictable. They become defensive. One day, for example, a patient in a treatment center where I was working shouted, "Hey, there are a *lot* of angry people around here." I made a quick appraisal of the people to whom he was referring: The physicians were doing fine, the nurses were getting along, the other staff were happy, and, for the most part, so were the rest of the patients. The fellow making the statement was the only angry human there! Projection is a defense mechanism that prevents us from looking at all the problems we don't want to deal with—the shadow side of ourselves. People who are sexually anorexic project onto others their sexual shadow side. They are very suspicious of their partner, for example, because they don't trust themselves.

All of us have different dimensions to our lives: work, love, sexuality, our families, our values, and so on. Part of our identity we make public; the rest we keep to ourselves. One ability healthy people have—a skill we all need—is to let other people know what's on our dark side. We don't open to just anyone, of course, and we shouldn't. But we should let some people inside. Why is this so important? By not acknowledging our shadow side, we actually give it greater strength, and eventually it will rise up and damage us. And, furthermore, denying our shadow side will prevent us from becoming who we really want to be.

I often play a little game with audiences to illustrate this point. I'll pick out someone, and say, "Okay, maybe one of the things you do is 'head switching.'" This means that when you look at two people who are sitting side by side, you switch their heads in your mind. Typically this isn't something one announces in front of other people—"I just looked at you guys and switched your heads, and you know, it was an improvement." No, it's best not to do that! But maybe at some point you decide to tell someone, and you say, "I want to tell you something about myself I've never told anybody, and sometimes it makes people angry when I do what I'm going to tell you about." You tell the person, and, after a long pause, the person replies, "Well, don't worry about it. You see, I've been head switching for years too. There are support groups for people like us!" Suddenly, you realize that you're not alone; others have this "problem" too.

Head switching is not, of course, a serious problem, but the example is nevertheless applicable to our concerns. The experience of the person who revealed the head-switching secret is a common one. When we acknowledge our dark side, just the act of doing so allows us to gain acceptance from others. At the same time, we also accept the part of ourselves that we've kept hidden. The result: Our dark side becomes a source of strength.

Let me once again return to the *Star Wars* story. Luke Skywalker's teachers, Obi-Wan Kenobi and Yoda, repeatedly cautioned him about the danger of being turned by the Dark Side. Here, the metaphor of the Dark Side refers to our not accepting our "humanness"—our human limitations. But Luke wanted to be more than he was or could be; he just couldn't accept his limitations. Life brings significant challenges that force us to face our human limitations; when we accept those limits—when we create appropriate boundaries for our lives—we are transformed.

Chapter 6 talked about the pain we can encounter on our healing journey. Part of this pain arises when we face and come to terms with our dark side. It's very much in the spirit of the Fourth Step of Twelve Step programs, which asks us to make a searching and *fearless* moral inventory of ourselves. It means we look squarely at *all* aspects of ourselves—including the parts we're embarrassed about or ashamed of—and then accept that we've done things that weren't very good for us.

Looking at and accepting our dark side allows us to at last integrate all sides of ourselves. We can begin to build on what we've seen and learned about ourselves. In treatment, for example, addicts are encouraged to see the positive aspects of their dark side. Perhaps they were very creative, persistent, or funny, or they had great sales skills (in dealing drugs!). In other words, even the qualities that nearly brought them down can, in recovery, become a source of strength.

We *must* discover and acknowledge what we see at the core of who we are, and when we do, we find that this is a profoundly informing place. We now have the ability to live with the strength of knowing who we are, what we can and can't do, what we're willing and unwilling to accept. In so doing, we become very different people when we enter relationships.

Self-Definition: Engaging the Spiritual

Acknowledging our dark side leads to and engages the second part of the self-definition process—the spiritual. When we find we can trust ourselves, we find, too, that we can also handle and be in any situation. When we are in passion, for example, we can let go and flow with it because we know we won't let ourselves be abused.

In this connection with who we are lies the first movement of a spiritual life. Henri Nouwen describes three major movements in spiritual growth.[2] The first is a connection with self— literally the transformation of loneliness into solitude. The mark of this transformation, he says, is the ability to be with one's self. It's a fundamental acceptance of who we are as individual human beings.

Once we can trust ourselves, the second movement follows naturally. We now assume that there are other people in the world whom we can trust. Not only do we see ourselves as worthwhile and trustworthy, but also we project that sense of worthiness to others. We are seen as a person of substance— someone who matters, who commands respect, and who will be respectful.

Once we trust ourselves and others, the final movement we must make is to trust our connection to something greater than ourselves, what is variously called the Higher Power, God, the One.

Here are Nouwen's own words:

> The difficult road is the road of conversion, the conversion from loneliness into solitude. Instead of running away from our loneliness and trying to forget or deny it, we have to protect it and turn it into a fruitful solitude. To live a spiritual life, we must first find the courage to enter into the desert of our loneliness and to change it by gentle and persistent efforts into a garden of solitude. This requires not only courage, but also a strong faith. As hard as it is to believe that the dry, desolate desert can yield endless varieties of flowers, it is equally hard to imagine that our loneliness is hiding unknown beauty. The movement from loneliness to solitude, however, is the beginning of any spiritual life because it is the movement from the restless senses to the inward-reaching search, from fearful clinging to fearless play.

Emptying ourselves of distractions, preoccupations, and obsessions allow us to connect with who we really are. It means discovering what German theologian Dietrich Bonhoeffer called "the ground of being." It is finding the sacred within us. When we are true to ourselves, we are most spiritual. We begin to tune to our own authentic voice.

How do we do that? Think of times in your life when, as you were about to do something, a little voice inside said, "Don't do this. If you do, there's going to be a bad ending." You heard the voice, but you ignored it and went right ahead and did whatever it was anyway. When things did turn out badly, you said to yourself, "I wish I would have listened to myself." Sound familiar?

Self-Definition

Here's what happened. Probably most of the other people around you seemed to trust that the situation would turn out for the best, and the other outside indicators said you should go ahead—so you felt you could disregard your inner voice. You didn't trust *yourself*, despite the fact that your instincts were absolutely right on. In such a situation, a loss of self occurs because you denied your voice. That voice is *you* speaking.

Jung spoke of a larger consciousness that we can tap into with our intuition—if we would but listen. This is called "discernment"—the ability to see clearly what is, especially in those situations when we have no rules, laws, or prior experience to direct us. This is where divine guidance and trusting ourselves meet.

When we regularly listen to our inner voice, others notice. People can quickly see that they are dealing with somebody of substance, somebody who knows what he or she believes and is willing to act on it. There's no false ego put up for others' inspection. What they see is what they get—and what they get is a truly authentic person.

People who listen to their inner voice are trustworthy. We may not always like what they say, but we know at a gut level that we like to be with them because we won't be blindsided, let down, or exploited.

Listening to and trusting our inner voice can be difficult because we often feel many pressures to ignore it. Yet trusting and listening to it are critical in developing our discernment. Knowing what and whom we can trust is one of the most critical human faculties that we have, second only, perhaps, to allowing other people to become close to us.

We all struggle with the issue of discernment. It often surfaces for me in situations with my children. Not so long ago, for example, one of my daughters was dating a drummer in a band. One day, she came to me and said, "Dad, the boys' van broke down. They have a gig in Chicago on Saturday, and we really need to use your van to carry their stuff. There's no other way we can get there!" I looked at her and said, "Where are *their* parents?" but apparently none of the other families had a truck or van.

At times like this, she could be a formidable adversary. "Look, none of the guys' parents have a van. You have a van, Dad, what's the resistance here?"

I thought, "Okay, when in doubt, use honesty." I answered, "All right, I'll tell you what I'm doing, but I don't think this will make sense to you. You see, I have this feeling, a voice that's telling me that if I let you have the van, we'll all be sorry."

She put her hands on her hips and said sarcastically, "So you have a *voice* in you that tells you you're going to be sorry if you do this? Reeeaaaally, Dad."

So I gave in. I told her to take the van, knowing that something was going to happen. She grabbed the keys and bounded happily out of the house, shouting, "Thanks, Dad. See you Sunday!"

And what happened? At some point in Chicago, they stopped for gas. The drummer was driving and my daughter got out to get the hose. Apparently the van was a bit too far from the pump, and he needed to back up a bit. The passenger door was still open, so when he gunned the engine and shot backwards, the door caught on the pump and ripped right off the van. Can you picture me looking out my front window as they pulled into my driveway with the door roped to the side of my van?

My daughter felt very bad about what had happened; I didn't need to say a word to her. In addition, though, I realized then that this whole incident wasn't completely about my daughter. I knew that every time I ignored my inner voice, I regretted it. I didn't listen to myself. I didn't trust myself quite enough, and so I received another lesson.

Author M. Scott Peck has a wonderful phrase in which he says, "Mental health is a commitment to reality at all times."[3] At some point, we finally allow ourselves to see that some parts of our lives simply aren't working. Living out of control sexually doesn't work. It creates chaos and damage for everyone involved. Shutting down sexually doesn't work, either. When we continue doing something that does not work, we've got a problem—a big problem. The real task, then, is to find a way to live in which we feel deeply satisfied and deeply congruent with our inner voice.

The closer we can get to this sense of clarity, the more we can stand up and be counted on for what matters; the greater sense of ourselves we have, the clearer life will be. *This* is what self-definition means. It is the linchpin that connects all we've looked at thus far in this book with all that's yet to come. Self-definition is absolutely critical. Professionals have put much effort into teaching people with sexual problems to trust others, to trust a process, to trust certain techniques. Our sexuality, however, is only tangentially affected by what others think or do. If we will only look closely enough, we will find that the problem is often within *us*: We lack the ability to trust ourselves. This ability is the cornerstone of our lives—including our healthy sexuality.

KEY QUESTIONS

Typically, in workshops and in my counseling experience, the following questions are asked in reference to self-definition.

How do I resolve tension between my sexual values and my sexual needs?

To resolve this dilemma, we must first answer the question: "Is it okay to have needs in the first place?" This issue was addressed earlier in the book, and particularly in chapter 6. Next we must look at our needs as they relate to our sexual selves, and then additional questions arise. What does it mean to be sexual, and do our needs and values mesh with this? We must first define ourselves as human beings: We must, in other words, define our goals, priorities, and values. Having done this, we can then turn our attention to our sexual values and ask ourselves if our values mesh with our sexual needs. I can imagine, for example, being sexual with many women. However, the reality of building a relationship with more than one woman is more than I can handle because of the tremendous attachment and importance I place on my relationships. If our sexual needs (and actions) are out of synch with our overall goals and values, sex will not feel fulfilling. Inner peace comes when our sexual expression is a part of that which gives us our greatest meaning.

Since my family was so crazy, how will I recognize appropriate sexual boundaries and how do I set them?
In healthy families, members experience and thus learn appropriate boundaries for sexual matters. But the many people who had no model for this truly do not know where to begin. In part, they don't know how to listen to their inner voice to find what feels right—in fact, they may actually be afraid to do so. We need to decide what gives us self-respect and meaning to our lives. We then link this value system with our needs and make them work together. Only then can we begin to determine boundaries that are appropriate for us.

ISSUES

Many sexual anorexics struggle with the following issues in reference to self-definition. Some of these issues have been explored at greater length in this or previous chapters; for those which have not, a brief discussion is included here. Read the issues carefully, noting the ones that apply to you. Then use those issues as discussion points with your partner and/or fair witnesses.

Self-Definition

❀ Experiencing the loss of self through deprivation.

❀ Having the inability to ask for personal needs to be met.

This speaks to the issue of knowing yourself; knowing both the no and the yes.

❀ Blaming others for sexual problems and failures.
One sign of distortion of self-definition is blaming others for our sexual problems and failures—it's about the husband, the ex-wife, the way I was raised, how men are and how women are, and so on. These efforts at blame serve only to distract us from looking for the real source of the problem.

❀ Having inadequate boundaries with others around sex, and feeling confused about values.
This issue is, of course, symptomatic of the loss of self and the confusion this brings. We should expect value conflict and confusion. This is part of the process—a process that leads us to ourselves, where we must confront our pain.

❀ Remaining "little" when one needs to be "full-sized" as a sexual person.
"Full-sized" women and men are grown-ups who take responsibility for themselves. They don't see their problems as the fault of other people. My inability to be orgasmic is not about you, it's about me and my orgasm. Children want to be taken care of and let adults make their decisions; "full-sized" people take responsibility for their *own* lives.

❀ Sending conflicting messages about sexuality to others because of internal inconsistencies.
If we're not consistent, we will give others in our lives double messages. Here's an example. Sue has an attraction for those of the same gender, but feels that she could never act on it. Her

relationships, however, operate with this pattern: "I'm really attracted to you, but when you get close, I pull back and leave." This stance confuses others because it's a message that says, "I'm interested, but I really will not pursue that option."

✳ Overcoming fearful, reluctant, and indecisive stances toward others.

This is the basic task we need to accomplish, and it stems from all the above issues. Though this is a critical developmental sexual task, it's not a complex one. If we're not able to take stands in general, we won't be able to do it when sex is involved. This task reflects the true spirit of the Fourth Step, which asks us to undertake courageous self-examination. It's an approach to mental health that says we want reality no matter what the cost. It's asking us to look directly at our real selves.

The Big Book of Alcoholics Anonymous says, "There are some of us who have cried out, 'This is too great a task.'" Certainly, this is a difficult task, but it is by no means too great. Many before us have accomplished it, and with the help of others, we can do likewise. Doing so is absolutely fundamental to this recovery process. Yet it is this very work—to have a realistic picture of who we are—that so many people fear and resist.

TASKS

Consider the following statements about self-definition and then complete the exercise that follows.

1. Many incentives exist for not taking a stand about who you are as a sexual person.
   If we like to avoid conflict, or if we don't deal well with feelings, not taking a stand is a good way to cope. Knowing who we are as people will help us take such a stand.

2. Obsession thrives in the unfinished and obscure difficult choices.

   Obsessive preoccupation is the fundamental component of sexual anorexia. When we are unable to make choices, we live constantly "in between," and it's this very fence-sitting that feeds obsession. Again, with a better idea of who we are, making decisions will become easier.

3. Jung's notion of "legitimate suffering" can be applied to sex. Real grief and pain do exist in people's lives. "Legitimate suffering" can be part of this experience, and through the recovery process, our suffering can become associated with what gives us meaning and can help clarify issues. We have tried to run from the pain long enough.

4. By clarifying sexual priorities and setting boundaries we can be safe and sexual.

   As suggested earlier, checking in with your support community and fair witnesses is so important. We need to break the no-talk rule about sexuality. Most of us believe that the only person we can talk to about sex is our partner—and even then we're very cautious. We need to be able, for example, to call someone and say, "You know, I have this thing that I think about sexually, and I want to know if you think it's really bad." We need to create and foster an openness about sexuality with our friends. To be able to talk freely about how things are going sexually is very relieving as well as a great help. We've just got to stop avoiding the sexual part of ourselves.

LOOKING AT YOUR SEXUAL DARK SIDE

This exercise is designed to help you begin looking at your sexual dark side by considering the questions listed below. Write your answers in your journal. In addition, share them with your partner and your fair witnesses.

1. What have you kept hidden in regard to your sexuality?

2. What have you not felt good about?

3. What matters to you sexually?

4. What sexual priorities do you have?

5. What concerns do you have about sexual safety?

6. What can you do to feel safe sexually?

PLANNING

Writing in your journal can help you cultivate discernment. In addition, develop a daily meditation routine, listen to music that makes you feel like yourself, and read books and magazines that help you develop your insight and sense of self. There is no magic about this process. If you work at it, your true voice—the one that is in harmony with the larger universe—will become clear.

IN YOUR JOURNAL

Start each morning by writing your "daily pages." Since this chapter focuses on self-definition, include thoughts about this topic in your journal. Write about your most important values. Write about your struggles with setting appropriate boundaries and taking responsibility for your actions. Write about your sexual values—how they have developed and changed.

A CLOSING EXERCISE

✐   The closing exercise asks you and your partner to evaluate yourselves and one another. Remember, this exercise offers a wonderful opportunity for you to discover your strengths and weaknesses, as well as a chance for you and your partner to compare your perceptions of yourselves and one another.

In addition to filling out the rating scales, it will be helpful to do the following:

- Once you have filled out your scales, share the results with your fair witnesses.
- After your partner has finished, talk about your partner's perceptions too. They may differ from yours and/or those of your fair witnesses.
- If significant discrepancies exist, note them and then return to your fair witnesses to look into them more carefully.

As you work on the scales, try not to become defensive if the perceptions your partner or your fair witnesses have of you differ from your own perceptions of yourself. Let these differences—and the reasons for them—be a source of information for all of you.

If you are not currently in a relationship, ask one of your fair witnesses (therapist, sponsor, anorexia group member, Twelve Step support group member, or RCA group member, for example) to work through the scales with you.

Part 1: Focus on You

On the first scale, consider your self-definition. Do you know what your values are? Can you set appropriate boundaries? Do you take responsibility for your actions? For your sexuality? How much work do you need on self-definition to feel comfortable with yourself?

Using a circle, rate yourself on the scale. (1 = low skills, need much work; 10 = high skills, need no further work.)

Next, ask your partner to rate you on self-definition. Have your partner use a square to rate you.

1   2   3   4   5   6   7   8   9   10

Part 2: Focus on Your Partner

On this second scale, ask your partner to consider his or her own self-definition. What are your partner's values? Can your partner set appropriate boundaries? Does your partner take responsibility for his or her actions? For his or her sexuality? How much work does your partner need on self-definition to feel comfortable?

Have your partner use a circle to rate himself or herself on self-definition.

Next, you rate your partner's skills and ability in this area. Use a square to do so.

I   2   3   4   5   6   7   8   9   10

Nurturing—
We learn to trust and to open our lives to experience.

Sensuality—
Through our senses, we interact with the world around us and become connected to it.

Self-Image—
We learn that we are good and lovable.

Self-Definition—
We develop a relationship with ourselves and come to trust ourselves. We are trustworthy.

10

SEXUAL COMFORT

polished not from love's steady partnership
you feel your way fluidly toward warm familiar
destinations inner pools unaware
you too have outgrown the need for armor

— Eileen Stratidakis

THE TERM *sexual comfort* is something of an oxymoron in a culture like ours where sexuality is either hidden and not talked about or distorted and used by corporations and the media as a selling tool for every conceivable product. Reaching even a minimal level of comfort about sexuality requires us to be open and willing to discuss the topic. And to talk about sex in a constructive, healthy manner requires breaking some rules about how we do that—which is exactly what I tell people who attend my workshops on sexuality.

Chapter 2 looked at intimacy and the kind of isolation and emotional constrictions that occur with sexual anorexia. Here it's important to be aware that to develop comfort with sexuality, we must work against very strong forces. These include centuries of religio-cultural imperatives against enjoying pleasure and sex, our modern-day culture's discomfort with sex and its no-talk rules, and our own inner resistance. We may also face a partner who is unwilling to aid our growth in sexual comfort and may even subvert our efforts.

The first task in becoming more comfortable with our sexuality is to notice and report our discomfort. What about sexuality do you find diffcult to read, or even think, about? When you and your partner are being intimate, do you feel irritated, become distracted, or wish to stop the process? By first paying attention to these feelings, and then taking time to talk with your partner and your fair witnesses about them, you can begin to see what lies at the root of your discomfort. You can begin to see areas in which you need to concentrate. And you can begin to work toward greater comfort.

As you read this chapter, pay close attention to the feelings you have about sex. Keep written notes about them, perhaps in your journal. Arrange to talk with your fair witnesses about them.

Again, it's important to recognize that increasing sexual comfort takes time and effort. In the Tasks section near the end of this chapter, you will find a list of highly recommended resources that can help you. Of particular help in beginning conversations about sexuality and sexual relationships, as well as for enhancing and revitalizing them, is *The Couples Comfort Book* by Jennifer Louden.

Sexual Embarrassment

If you were sitting in the audience at one of my workshops, I might ask you to pause and remember an embarrassing sexual incident from your past. Stop and take a moment to do so now, and then read ahead for one of my own favorites.

During my fifth-grade year, I was at a party with friends, and at some point during the evening, we decided to play spin the bottle. For a bunch of uptight Lutheran and Catholic kids, believe me, this was quite an accomplishment! I'd never kissed a girl before, so I was mighty nervous about playing this game!

When my turn came, I spun the bottle, and it pointed at a girl named Cheryl. "My God!," I thought, because to me Cheryl was one of the prettiest girls in our whole grade. Okay, I had to kiss her, so I closed my eyes and . . . I missed her mouth completely, landing that kiss squarely on her eye instead! You can imagine the uproar that created! Everyone there, of course, saw me kiss Cheryl on the eye. By second hour the next morning at school, *everyone* knew about my kissing Cheryl on the eye. Today, this is one of those youthful moments I look back on and chuckle about, but at the time, I was *so* embarrassed.

We have *all*, of course, had such moments, and it can be fun to think about them. However, we need to be aware of how much shame we felt about these situations, which, in turn, kept us from ever talking to anyone about them.

Now that you're thinking about your sexual history, here's another task. Think about the messages on sexuality you received from your family as you grew up. I still clearly remember the lecture my father gave me on masturbation—the content of which he had gleaned from the U.S. Army during World War II! He basically told me that every time a man masturbates (of course, he said nothing about women doing this), he loses an amount of starch from his body equivalent to having hiked seven miles. This just didn't seem believable to me, because, after a quick calculation, I figured that at the rate I was going, I should have been crippled! The message, of course, was that masturbation is bad for you.

Families create many rules about sexuality. "We don't talk about it," for instance. Rules about what's okay for boys, but not for girls. Or "If you do it, we don't want to hear about it." Or "Everybody's sexual business is public and everybody in the family knows about what everybody is doing," even though this is inappropriate. Rules may be in the form of double messages, such as parents saying fidelity is important while one or both are having multiple affairs. Family rules and boundaries about touch cover a broad spectrum too. In some families, public displays of affection are seen as inappropriate; in others, incestuous relationships occur.

We find ourselves as a society caught in a difficult situation. Today, with sexually transmitted diseases occurring at epidemic rates, the deadly threat of AIDS, and sexual activity among teens at very high levels, it's more important than ever that everyone have good information about sexuality. We simply can't afford the kind of ignorance many of us grew up with.

But how do we accomplish this task? Many people believe that teaching about sexuality rightfully belongs to the family, as do I. Yet at the same time, study after study shows that parents simply aren't doing the job. And that shouldn't be surprising because in most cases, *their* parents never taught them about sexuality—or they received the equivalent of my father's masturbation speech. How can parents teach their children well if they aren't educated about sex themselves, and if they are deathly afraid to even discuss the matter? Compounding the problem, when schools try to step into the picture, they get clobbered by parents and churches for interfering.

Another major childhood influence on sexual attitudes is religion—the next area I explore with my audiences. What messages did you receive from your pastor, church, or religious schools?

My first experience in this area was in the confessional. Sadly, I was sexually abused by a neighbor woman when I was just three and a half years old—an experience that had enormous and very long-lasting implications for me. When I was six, and thus old enough to go to confession, I told the priest about the abuse I'd suffered. This actually turned out to be a positive experience for me because, after listening to my story, he said, "Well, was this woman a grown-up?" and, of course, she was. The message I took home from the church that day was that this wasn't my fault—and as a child, I *had*, of course, thought the opposite.

Virtually all abuse survivors labor under a similarly false and often destructive assumption. I was tremendously relieved by what I'd heard, and my sexual healing actually began within the context of the church. While many people receive unhelp-ful messages about their sexuality in their religious upbringing, I want to stress that clergy and churches can and do have pos-itive as well as negative effects on their congregations.

I have had the opportunity to speak to many, many people about sexual comfort, and what I most often notice about audiences is that they will only reluctantly begin talking about this topic. But by the time we've begun exploring religious influences, they've usually become so involved that I nearly have to shout to stop the conversations.

Identifying Our Discomforts

Working to become more comfortable and open about our sexuality is very difficult in a culture that's anything but com-fortable with the subject, especially if we have suffered sexually in some way. Moving ahead with this task supports our efforts in self-definition because once we "put our arms around" and share with others both the dark and light side of our sexuality, we become far more comfortable with it.

In many ways, this process resembles the Fifth Step of Alcoholics Anonymous, "We admitted to God or our Higher Power, to ourselves, and to another person the exact nature of our wrongs"—and when we were wronged. These are jour-neys of profound self-honesty shared with another—and once we are accepted by another, acceptance of self takes place too. These experiences can be deeply spiritual, in that we find acceptance at a level beyond our greatest expectations.

Many, many people find that they feel greatly relieved when they at last break the wall of silence surrounding sex. It can feel so good to finally let go and talk about all this. We are, after all, sensual, sexual beings, and remaining silent about sex, bottling up all our opinions and feelings and concerns and questions, takes a lot of energy. What's more, depending on what we're keeping inside, the effects can have unforeseen consequences, as happened to me a few years ago.

While preparing for a Public Broadcasting System (PBS) series on addiction, I decided it would be a good idea to get some professional "tutoring" on how to present myself on television. I had already participated in general media training—learning how to field questions and deal with difficult reporters, for instance—but handling my own program, as I would be expected to do, takes more work.

Among other things, the television coach with whom I worked showed me how to get down into a funny kind of crouch that makes people look good on camera when they're standing. Unfortunately, it's an awkward and clumsy position to be in, and I decided I needed to practice it whenever possible. Presenting at my own workshops seemed to offer the perfect opportunity for this, so I did. When I was up in front of my audience, I'd walk around in this odd crouch, and invariably someone would ask what I was doing. I'd tell them the story—that I was preparing for television and I had to strengthen my muscles.

After a couple of weeks, however, my thighs and buttocks started to hurt. It soon became bad enough that I began to wonder if the television program were worth all this pain. A very dear friend recommended a reliable massage therapist. I made an appointment, and, upon arriving, told the therapist about the pain in my legs and buttocks. The therapist asked me to be very specific about where the pain was, and, as soon as I described it, the therapist said, "Are you a sexual abuse victim?"

That was one of those moments when the light goes on and immediately a host of seemingly disparate events fall together. In this case, I immediately realized that it would be in the PBS series that I'd first publicly talk about my sexual abuse experiences as a child. It's not unusual for abuse survivors to hold the muscles around their anus and genitals tight as a way of protecting themselves—and, as a result, their legs and buttocks become sore because of the muscle spasms. I knew this could happen, yet I was oblivious to it. What I had thought to be a problem with the crouch was instead about an abuse issue and my terrible discomfort in talking about it, especially on national television. When the therapist asked that question, what was really going on became obvious to me.

After I answered yes to the question, the massage therapist then launched into a lecture about what a survivor of abuse can do to help with muscles that have tightened like this. It was a lecture that *I* had given many times—but now it was happening to me!

Though this example is perhaps a bit extreme, the point is nevertheless well taken. What we don't get into the open and deal with will affect us sooner or later—even though we're oblivious to the anxiety it's creating. We need to identify our "discomforts" because they will, in fact, sneak up on us and catch us unaware, sometimes when we are the most vulnerable.

Talking with Our Partner

When I talk about sexual comfort, I mean the capacity to be at ease about sexual matters with ourselves and with others—being at ease with our own sexuality and having the ability to talk about sexual matters with our partner—and with other trusted people in our lives, as well. Sexual health is very much connected to sexual communication. As stated in chapter 7, Masters and Johnson believed that in order for sex to work, partners need to talk before, during, and after sex. Sexual communication is perhaps the most critical part of what takes place within a couple—far more so than their genitals or physical attraction and the rest. It's simply critical to be able to communicate about what's going on with each other.

Many couples run into difficulty because partners do not take time to tell each other their fears, worries, wants, needs, and desires. Without good communication, huge misunderstandings can develop and interfere substantially with the partners' ability to be sexual with one another.

A problem can start quite innocently, based on a simple

assumption such as "When you do this, I think it means such and such." A classic example plays out as follows. Helen's thinking: "If I'm not sexual, Paul will leave me, so I have to be sexual even though I don't want to be." Over time, she builds up an obsessional pattern, constantly worrying: "Is he going to ask me to do this again?" At the same time, Paul's thinking that it doesn't feel very good to him to be sexual with someone who doesn't want to be sexual with him—*and* who *says* she wants to be sexual but really doesn't. He then begins to worry: "Helen doesn't want to be sexual with me because I'm not satisfying her, and that must mean there's something wrong with what I'm doing." Both Helen and Paul are operating under erroneous assumptions generated and maintained simply because they're not talking to each other. This is exactly how the obsessional nature of sexual anorexia and sexual addiction is unwittingly fed within couples.

This example, and hundreds more, demonstrate how critical it is to really talk about sex. Too many people have the unfortunate and mistaken impression that talking about sex will somehow destroy its spontaneity and/or passion. On the contrary, it's not talking that's getting in the way!

Sex, after all, is one of the great acts of communication. But many couples go about it in a silent and perfunctory way. This routinization of sex is sure to dampen the fire! Partners need to learn to express their feelings and emotions during sex. When something feels good, let your partner know. When partners remain silent and nonexpressive, this can cause doubt as to whether they are really enjoying themselves physically. Expressing pleasure through words or sounds signals to your partner that you are enjoying yourself. This will lead to increased arousal for both of you. Once the juices are flowing, let the sounds of pleasure well up and express themselves! The results can be terrific.

Partners need to sit down and discuss what's going on between them sexually. Passion and spontaneity flow from the wellspring of self, not from the demands of another. Partners need to ask: What really does this mean? What does this feel like? Do you like this? Do you want that?

Communication not only includes expressing pleasure during sex, but also letting your partner know afterwards just what seemed to work. Couples can go for years without telling one another what excites them. That's so unfortunate when a simple word here or there, or even a demonstration, can make a huge difference. If you really like oral stimulation of your clitoris, then let your partner know. If you love it when she climbs on top of you, then tell her. That way, you can keep the fires burning.

By opening up to each other, over time partners can become comfortable with their own and each other's sexuality. Once each partner's needs, desires, and fears are in the open, their worries and assumptions put to rest, the door opens wide for great spontaneity and passion because both partners can finally relax and play.

Talking with Others

This second aspect of sexual communication and comfort—being able to talk about our sexuality with people other than our partner—can be more difficult than communicating with our partner, but it's no less important. And here's yet another way we can break the no-talk rule about sex. Virtually all of us either are now or have been in a romantic and sexual relationship. Yet when we get together with good friends or in a support group, how often is the topic of our sexuality mentioned? And, if it does come up, what are the conversations like? Too often, I suspect, we merely complain about our frustrations with our partner—"He'd rather hunt or watch sports than be with me!" or "She's always 'too tired.' " Talking isn't the only problem; in fact, it may not even be the primary one. *How* we talk about sex is at least as important an issue. Clearly, we all think about, have questions about, and struggle with sex. It's talking about sex in a way that can actually help us become more satisfied with our experiences that is so important and badly needed.

Sex doesn't have to be such a secret topic. Once we begin sharing this part of ourselves, we find it becomes easier and more comfortable. Those we talk with often react with relief too. What do we fantasize about? What's been getting in the way of sex for us? What do we like? Dislike? Struggle with? When we talk about sex, we find that others have similar experiences and concerns. We and our friends and fair witnesses can learn from one another. We can support one another.

Over time, talking about sex can feel natural and easy. I have been meeting a couple of times a year with a group of therapists since 1986, and it's been a very supportive gathering for all of us. Many of the women in our group are now menopausal, so frank discussions about what menopause is like are common. There's an ease with which we talk about this topic that's helpful—and fun, too—for all of us. In addition, it's provided me with a perspective on my relationship with my spouse.

The benefits of learning to accept our sexuality—to know and share who we are as sexual beings—go beyond relationships with partner and friends. The feelings of shame and disgust our culture carries about sexuality can and do endanger and hurt all of us. At the beginning of the AIDS epidemic, for example, when it had finally become clear that AIDS was going to have a worldwide impact, the British government decided it needed to learn more about people's sexual behavior. Believing such information would be critical for controlling the nascent epidemic, the government commissioned a study of sexual behavior in the United Kingdom.

As with any government-funded scientific study, an approval process was undertaken. All the scientists involved strongly supported the study. At some point, however, it attracted public attention. Once that happened, then-Prime Minister Margaret Thatcher canceled the project, saying that it was unnecessary and that private, personal information about the British people simply didn't need to be studied or publicized. This is a classic example of how we as a culture cannot talk about or deal with sexual issues—with costly and disastrous consequences for many people.

KEY QUESTIONS

Typically, in workshops and in my counseling experience, the following question is asked when we talk about sexual comfort.

No matter what I try, I have never been totally comfortable about sex. Why? What happens if my mother was right about sex?
Remember, first, that whatever we learned about sexuality has been with us for a long time, so the changes in attitude I'm suggesting are significant—and the transformation won't happen overnight. Now that we've identified the direction in which we want to go, we need to focus on trying to move a little bit closer to our goal each day. If someone had told me in the 1970s, for example, that someday I would stand in front of an audience of hundreds and talk about masturbation, I'd have tried to get the person certified as insane. I have now done this many times, but it didn't happen suddenly. I can look back and see how much I've changed.

All of us can make these changes. There's no secret, no trick. Look to and talk with your fair witnesses, friends, partner, support group, whomever. Just begin, and before long, you'll find yourself with a level of comfort about sexuality that you never thought possible.

ISSUES

Many sexual anorexics struggle with the following issues in reference to sexual comfort. Some of these issues have been explored at greater length in this or previous chapters; for those which have not, a brief discussion is included here. Read the issues carefully, noting the ones that apply to you. Then use those issues as discussion points with your partner and/or fair witnesses.

❀ Having a limited history of being at "ease" with sex.

❀ Overcoming negative religious messages about sex.

❀ Facing dysfunctional parental and cultural rules about sex.

❀ Understanding obsession as a way to avoid the pain and joy of sex.

Sexual anorexics say they want nothing to do with sex, don't want to be reminded about sex, don't even want to talk about it. They are, however, extremely preoccupied with sex. Here obsession has become a tool to ease anxiety.

If we can lower anxiety in another, more healthy way, then obsession will dissolve. What lowers anxiety? Increasing our sexual comfort, of course! And with the anxiety gone, there's no longer a payoff for maintaining the obsession.

I can't overemphasize the importance of talking about sex and developing sexual comfort. Obsession has a hard time surviving when it's no longer a secret. Revealing obsession is like putting mold in sunlight. It dries up and withers away. When we talk to others about such issues, we quickly realize they're more common than we thought—and not so formidable, either. The more people we talk to about sexuality, the more comfortable we become. Being at ease talking with our partner *and* others about sexuality is one of the basic components of healthy sexuality.

Sexual Comfort

🦋 Confronting issues of sexual orientation.

Two dimensions come into play in this issue. When we discussed self-definition in the previous chapter, we didn't really examine what happens when that self-definition runs contrary to what many people believe to be normal. Gays, lesbians, and bisexuals face a more complicated challenge in the area of sexual comfort. Talking about sexual orientation, for example, might not only be uncomfortable, but also it could have serious personal and professional ramifications. Listen as Carl, a thirty-six-year-old gay man, describes his ongoing journey of self-definition.

> We clearly live in a society in which few people talk about sex to begin with. For gay and lesbian children, the little that's heard about sex is, of course, only about heterosexual sex. Generally there's no talk about gay sex in a home, unless a parent is gay or the family is open enough to know gays or lesbians and includes them in the family's social circle. That wasn't my experience, however.
>
> As a young child growing up in Cleveland in the 1970s, I was teased a lot, especially in sixth and seventh grades—I guess because I just wasn't a typical guy—not competitive, not a good athlete, and so on. In high school, I was fairly popular, especially with women. I was someone they could talk to, I wasn't a jerk, and I wasn't always coming on to them.
>
> In high school, I came across as being sort of disinterested in sex, almost asexual. Other kids didn't ask me much about dating because, I think, everyone was uncomfortable with the idea of my going out with girls. When I was older, some of my high school friends did tell me they wondered at the time if I was gay. I wasn't teased much at all in high

school, perhaps because I was physically mature and pretty muscular. I was fortunate in a way, because people left me alone.

On the other hand, I also felt extremely alone and isolated. I just really didn't know about being gay. I knew I was more attracted to men, but no one ever told me you could be sexual with someone of the same gender. I didn't know it was a possibility. I thought I was the only one who had these feelings. I didn't really even know what homosexuality was!

So, of course, I had no one to talk to about being gay, and the little I knew about it came from a bit of reading I did. Here, however, the message given was that gays were men who really just wanted to be women. I puzzled over that a lot because I didn't think that was what I felt. I didn't want to be a woman. This might be an issue for some people who do want to change gender, but that is NOT what gay men want. Today I can say that I enjoy being a man, and I want to make love with another man.

Once I figured out what was going on with me, I had huge amounts of shame about being gay. I was even more lonely, and I internalized a lot of negative feelings. I had absolutely no homosexual role models, and I just felt really alone and completely without knowledge.

After graduating from high school, I left Cleveland to go to college in Minneapolis-St. Paul, in part because there was a good school in the area, but also because there was a good-sized gay community.

Once there, I became part of the gay culture. My coming-out process began. Coming out really has a lot to do with joining the gay culture. For me, as for many gay men, this brings an end to our isolation. Another thing that helped me a lot was getting involved in gay organizations in college. For the first time in my life, I had some gay friends—gays my own age with whom I could socialize. At long last I began to find some comfort with myself as a gay person.

I can see now that for some years, I ghettoized myself in the gay community. It's where I was really comfortable, and I pretty much stayed there once I found it. But I did need to find out who I was—this was very much related to my self-image and self-definition—who I was as a person was for the first time supported by others. Sometimes gays are criticized for ghettoizing, but for me this time was a buffer against the abuse we all get in the straight world. I really needed this time with other gay men.

I need to stress, too, that coming out is something that takes place over time; it doesn't just happen once at a certain age. Gays are hidden in many ways in this culture. We don't wear our gender preference on our shirt sleeves, so to speak. There's always the assumption that we're heterosexual. Our sexual preference is not immediately visible like race is, for instance. Gayness can be private or shared, and whether you do share it depends on how important it is to do so. In addition, there are many closets to come out of: you have to come out to yourself, to your community, to your family (if you can; some gays never do this), and also to the general world. Coming out is a process that goes on all your life.

A good example of this happened just the other day. I was driving my partner Stephen's car to work, and the guys I work with asked where the car came from. Now here's a very simple question, which would be nothing for a straight person to answer. For me as a gay guy to answer truthfully has enormous ramifications. In that split second, I had to decide—and gays have to do this all the time—how much of who I am I want to reveal. You always wonder how someone will react when you tell them. I said the car was my partner Stephen's. Not knowing I was gay until that moment, there was a lot of murmuring—but no problems thus far.

✻ Resolving issues generated by sexual abuse.
Resolving issues generated by sexual abuse requires looking into our dark side and being able to say, "Well, yes, that's what happened," and bringing this to resolution—in other words, finding our place of comfort with ourselves and our lives.

In her excellent book on healing from sexual abuse, *The Sexual Healing Journey*, author and psychotherapist Wendy Maltz describes Lynn's experience as a twenty-seven-year-old married survivor.

> Sexual healing is a dynamic process. We gain understanding about how our sexuality has been affected by sexual abuse, make changes in our sexual attitudes and behaviors, and develop new skills for experiencing sex in a positive way. One type of change encourages another.
>
> When Lynn was a child, her older brother would often take her in the bathroom, fondle her, and attempt intercourse with her. Years later, Lynn married her high school sweetheart, Hal. Throughout their marriage, Lynn had difficulty becoming sexually aroused and enjoying sex. Sex

became rare and was often an upsetting ordeal.

Before Lynn sought counseling, she had no idea that her sexual problems with Hal might have resulted from the earlier sexual abuse. It wasn't until Lynn wept uncontrollably after sex one night that she realized a serious problem existed and that she needed help. While in counseling, Lynn made a connection between her ongoing sexual problems and the molestation by her brother. She discovered that she had learned to view sex as a duty, an act without choice, and an experience strongly associated with vaginal pain. Her sexual withdrawal from Hal was related to her old fears.

This new understanding prompted Lynn to begin changing her attitudes about sex. Lynn wondered if what she thought was sex was really sex abuse. She began to feel she had been cheated out of learning that sex could be something desirable, pleasurable, and fun. And she realized she could be a sexually healthy person after all.

With the help of counseling, Lynn learned a new skill. She learned to create a temporary moratorium on sex, giving her needed time to heal and helping her realize she had a choice to say no to her husband's sexual advances. Lynn stopped associating sex with obligation, guilt, and pressure. She spent months learning to initiate and enjoy nonsexual touch. With Hal's cooperation, she did special exercises to relax and stretch her vaginal muscles to make intercourse more comfortable. Lynn worked intensively for more than a year, and slowly she understood and resolved her feelings about the abuse.

As Lynn practiced her new skill, she experienced her sexual feelings in a new way. her responses changed. Eventually, Lynn's sexual experiences came to feel within her control and for her own pleasure.

"I didn't know what "sexual person" meant before. To allow myself to become sexually aroused has been a wonderful learning experience. I'm still learning to deal with sexual feelings . . . not to turn them off, but to let them grow and become more sexual. I can just hug Hal if I want to do that, or make love, if that's what both of us feel like doing. If it's not right, I can say so. I've never felt like I had these choices before."

It is possible to begin a sexual healing journey. We can identify our sexual concerns, learn how sexual abuse has affected our sexuality, get rid of old attitudes and behaviors that resulted from the abuse, and develop a new, healthier approach to sexual enjoyment. [1]

The stories of Carl and Lynn depict areas of sexual conflict and are examples of how people can achieve sexual comfort.

TASKS

The topic of sex produces anxiety on its own without all the added baggage from family and culture. Obsession has for many been a way to duck the central anxieties of sexuality, and change requires coming to terms with these fears.

The following exercises will help you move toward greater sexual comfort.

AN EMBARRASSING SEXUAL INCIDENT

1. Think back to an embarrassing sexual incident that happened to you. Describe it in your journal.

2. Talk about this incident with your partner, spouse, or fair witnesses. Consider the following questions when doing so.

   - How did you feel at the time of the incident?

   - How do you feel today about it?

   - If there is a difference, how did that change come about?

   - What does this say about your sexual comfort level today?

FAMILY RULES

1. Families create many rules about sexuality. Try to remember as many of your family's messages as you can, and write them in your journal.

2. Talk about these rules with your partner, spouse, or fair witnesses. Consider the following questions when doing so.

   - Was it difficult to identify these rules? If so, why?

   - What effects have these rules had on you and your relationships?

   - Which of these rules would you "rewrite," and what would the new rules say?

RELIGIOUS RULES

1. Many of us learn rules about sexuality from the teachings of our religion. Try to remember some of the religious-based rules you learned, and write them in your journal.

2. Talk about these rules with your partner, spouse, or sponsor. Consider the following questions when doing so.

   - Was it difficult to identify these rules? If so, why?

   - What effects have these rules had on you and your relationships?

   - Which of these rules would you "rewrite," and what would the new rules say?

RESOURCES FOR SEXUAL COMMUNICATION

Here are some excellent resources for enhancing your ability to communicate with others about sex. Try to obtain a copy of one or more of the following books. Share what you learn with your partner and/or fair witnesses.

- *The Couples Comfort Book: A Creative Guide for Renewing Passion, Pleasure and Commitment* by Jennifer Louden

- *The Sexual Healing Journey: A Guide for Survivors of Sexual Abuse* by Wendy Maltz

- *Allies in Healing: When the Person You Love Was Sexually Abused as a Child* by Laura Davis

- *Hot Monogamy: Essential Steps to More Passionate, Intimate Lovemaking* by Patricia Love and Jo Robinson

- *Joyous Sexuality: Healing from the Effects of Family Sexual Dysfunction* by Mic Hunter

PLANNING

In addition to the above exercises, get together, if possible, with each of the people who have been part of this healing journey with you thus far. Explore the following:

- Which issues have been easy to examine and deal with, and which have been more difficult?

- Note what each of those involved find easy and difficult, and talk about the differences and similarities.

- How has going through this process affected each of those people? Has it affected their relationships too? If so, in what ways?

IN YOUR JOURNAL

Begin each morning by writing your "daily pages." In addition, since this chapter focuses on sexual comfort, include thoughts about this topic in your journal. Here are some suggestions: How has your level of sexual comfort changed over the years? What areas do you find difficult to talk about or address? What are your goals in regard to this aspect of sexuality?

A CLOSING EXERCISE

✐   The closing exercise asks you and your partner to evaluate yourselves and one another. Remember, this exercise offers a wonderful opportunity for you to discover your strengths and weaknesses, as well as a chance for you and your partner to compare your perceptions of yourselves and one another.

In addition to filling out the rating scales, it will be helpful to do the following:

- Once you have filled out your scales, share the results with your fair witnesses.
- After your partner has finished, talk about your partner's perceptions too. They may differ from yours and/or those of your fair witnesses.
- If significant discrepancies exist, note them and then return to your fair witnesses to look into them more carefully.

As you work on these scales, try not to become defensive if the perceptions your partner or your fair witnesses have of you differ from your own perceptions of yourself. Let these differences—and the reasons for them—be a source of information for all of you.

If you are not currently in a relationship, ask one of your fair witnesses (therapist, sponsor, anorexia group member, Twelve Step support group member, or RCA group member, for example) to work through the scales with you.

Part 1: Focus on You

On the first scale, consider your level of sexual comfort. Can you and do you talk to your partner about your sexual desires? Can and do you talk with others besides your partner about sexuality? How much work do you need on sexual comfort?

Patrick Carnes

Using a circle, rate yourself on the scale. (1 = low skills, need much work; 10 = high skills, need no further work.)

Next, ask your partner to rate your sexual comfort. Have your partner use a square to rate you.

1   2   3   4   5   6   7   8   9   10

Part 2: Focus on Your Partner

On this second scale, ask your partner to consider sexual comfort as it applies to him or her. Can your partner talk to you about his or her sexual desires? Does your partner do this? Can and does your partner talk with others besides you about sexuality? How much work does your partner need on sexual comfort?

Have your partner use a circle to rate himself or herself.

Next, you rate your partner on sexual comfort. Use a square to do so.

1   2   3   4   5   6   7   8   9   10

Nurturing—
We learn to trust and to open our lives to experience.

Sensuality—
Through our senses, we interact with the world around us and become connected to it.

Self-image—
We learn that we are good and lovable.

Self-definition—
We develop a relationship with ourselves and come to trust ourselves. We are trustworthy.

Comfort—
We learn that we can trust others.

11

KNOWLEDGE

Healthy sexual relating is a lifelong journey.
It's a mystery we unlock through our own experiences
—Wendy Maltz

ONE OF THE MOST REMARKABLE CHANGES we've seen in our culture in the last three decades is the explosion of classes and educational programs geared specifically for adult learners. Countless opportunities exist now for adults who want to further their education. Classes cover a broad spectrum, ranging from a focus on specific skills such as knitting or welding to advanced degree programs at colleges and universities. Adult education programs—offered at high schools, community education centers, vocational-technical schools, community colleges, and universities—flourish for the simple reason that adults want them and are prepared to commit precious time and energy to reach their goals. All of us know adults who've taken up new avocations or changed careers. When people have a strong interest in some area—be it about their career or child rearing or music or first aid, or whatever—they find the time and energy to learn about it.

What I have found particularly curious, however, is that despite the interest most everyone has in sexuality, *very* few people put any energy into learning more about it. Why this is so is difficult to discern, but perhaps the reason is rooted in our society-wide no-talk rule about sex. Can you imagine course offerings such as "Making Your Sex Life More Interesting" or "Fantasize for Better Sex" or "Improving Your Sex Life after Age 40" in your local community education program?! Do you think anyone would sign up even if such classes were offered?

No, too many Americans view sexuality as something they should learn about on their own in private. Making any formal effort to learn more about our sexuality could mean we are, at best, a little odd, if not downright weird or perverted.

You might pause for a moment and think about your experience buying this book. What feelings did you have about buying it? Were you wondering what the salesclerk was thinking about you? Was the clerk wondering why you wanted the book? Was it for a friend or for you? Did you walk around with the book in your hand, or in a bag? Is this book kept in a place in your home where a friend or neighbor could run across it, or is it tucked away someplace "safe"—out of sight, in other words?

Clearly, a difference exists between what we need and want to know about sexuality, and what we actually take the time and effort to learn. By buying this book, however, you did take a step to learn more, and let me congratulate you now for what you're doing. You decided not only that you wanted to know more about your sexuality, but also that you would take action. You're working to try to understand and learn more, and you deserve a good deal of credit for that—both because you'll help yourself, and because you're making a contribution to the larger culture by chipping away at the no-talk rule.

A tremendous amount of accurate, clear, helpful, nonjudgmental information about human sexuality geared specifically to the general public is finally available today. (See the back of this book for a recommended list of resources.)

This chapter focuses on two very important areas, the human sexual response cycle and the role of sexual fantasy.

Knowing more about these topics will greatly enhance your understanding of human sexuality.

The Human Sexual Response Cycle

The human sexual response cycle has four phases: arousal, plateau, orgasm, and resolution. The *arousal phase* is characterized by initial attraction and interest and by feelings of sexual desire. As these feelings increase, we reach the *plateau phase*. Here, the level of arousal becomes sustained in preparation for achieving an orgasm. This phase can be long or short, but eventually it builds to a point at which orgasm is possible. The *orgasm phase* is usually brief, but it's the most intense part of the cycle. After orgasm comes the *resolution phase*, during which our sexual system returns to a nonaroused state. Many people describe feeling an "afterglow" and a sense of well-being as the body moves back to a normal state of being.

The human sexual response cycle varies from person to person, as well as from time to time for a given individual. A woman masturbating, for example, may one time find her arousal very quick, with a brief plateau, an intense orgasm, and a short resolution. On another occasion, this same woman might find that her arousal takes a long time, with a protracted plateau, no orgasm, and a long period of resolution. During intercourse with her spouse, she might experience a prolonged arousal, but then a short plateau followed by a very intense orgasm and a longer resolution period. This woman could have these varied experiences over just a few days.

If we pay attention, we will notice that our own sexual response cycle does have general patterns. It's important to know this occurs so that as we experience the different patterns, we can work within them to make a given sexual experience more pleasurable and fulfilling. Furthermore, it's equally important to know our partner's patterns, too, so the mutual experiences can be more pleasurable and fulfilling.

Knowing more about our arousal patterns can also provide

critical information about blocks in our sexual response cycle and how they relate to past experiences. There are two levels of knowledge: (1) how our bodies actually work physiologically, and (2) how we can work within our own response cycle to make sex work better for us.

FRANCINE'S STORY

The experiences of a woman I'll call "Francine" provide an excellent example of the benefits of understanding one's sexual response cycle. As a child, Francine found she very much liked to masturbate and, in fact, did—so much so that her masturbation caused trouble for her. She masturbated frequently enough at school in first and second grade that she was actually caught and sent home for it on several occasions. When this happened, Francine felt publicly humiliated, but still she couldn't stop. Francine was growing up in a family in which there was a great deal of tension, and masturbating was a way for her to relieve that tension. Unfortunately, however, Francine continued to be quite afraid of getting caught.

When Francine was twelve years old, her parents divorced and she went to live with her father. During the next couple of years, there were times when Francine's father would have her sleep in his bed. Though he never overtly or sexually touched her, he nevertheless laid against her. Francine was very frightened by these experiences, and felt clearly violated by them.

When she became an adult, Francine found her life characterized by a series of degrading and abusive relationships in which the sex was always quite intense. Francine eventually sought treatment for chemical addiction and codependency. In addition, she began looking at some of the other issues in her life that seemed to trouble her, and she finally had the opportunity to turn her attention to her sexual response cycle. In doing so, Francine noticed that she didn't have much trouble in the arousal phase—she was attracted to men, she felt desire, and she became aroused. But sustaining that arousal—the plateau phase—was another story. At this point in the cycle, Francine would find herself becoming scared, and then she'd begin to shut down.

In her work with her therapist, it became apparent to Francine that throughout her history with men, indeed going back to those experiences with her father, she feared that she would not be able to protect herself if she ever really let herself be open and vulnerable. During sex, Francine would find herself blocked and shutting down as soon as she felt unsafe, and that would always happen during the plateau phase. If Francine got past the plateau phase, orgasm would not be a problem—but staying in the plateau was very difficult. Eventually, Francine came to understand that in this stage we are very open and vulnerable—and it was these feelings that brought back all her fears—feeling vulnerable was frightening, not pleasurable.

In the resolution phase, Francine found herself with another problem—after she had an orgasm, everything stopped. She went cold and didn't want to have anything to do with the man she was with. It was as though someone had turned off the switch and slammed the door to her feelings.

Francine eventually realized that this response was connected to her experiences as a child when she was caught masturbating. Part of what we learn when we masturbate is to experience the lingering feelings of the resolution phase, the gentle waves of pleasure that continue to course through our bodies after orgasm. Because of her fear of being caught masturbating, Francine learned instead to shut herself down immediately after orgasm—staying calm and relaxed, letting feelings linger, just wasn't safe.

In examining her sexual response cycle, Francine thus discovered two distinct times when she was vulnerable. (See figure II.I.) In addition to this discovery, Francine found that it was a tremendous breakthrough to be able to talk about this situation and her fears with her new partner. This man, together with Francine's therapist and other friends who supported her, helped Francine see that she was no longer a helpless little girl; she was an adult woman who was more than capable of taking care of herself in a trusting relationship. Francine at last realized that her fears were now unwarranted.

To get past her problems, Francine first needed to learn more about how her response cycle operated physiologically. She was then able to determine exactly where her blocks were occurring. Having this knowledge made it possible for Francine—with the help of supportive friends and some professional help—to delve into previous relationships and her childhood to find the roots of her difficulties—and eventually overcome them. Francine is now in a three-plus year relationship in which both she and her partner are very happy.

Figure 11.1   A Sample Sexual Response Cycle

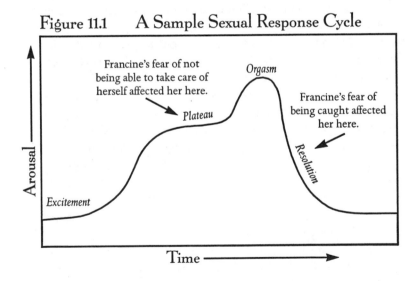

Gaining Knowledge and Preparing for Change

In the previous chapters, we focused on looking at ourselves, accepting who we are, and then moving on to developing greater levels of comfort with our sexuality. Here we are primarily focusing on gaining knowledge—about ourselves and our sexuality—to prepare ourselves for greater change and growth.

Classic Twelve Step language refers to this as removing our character defects, but here we talk about identifying areas on which we want to work. We've accepted who we are now, so our next Step, Step Six, is to think about the kind of person we want to become. In what ways can we improve ourselves? Step Six requires us to be completely honest with ourselves as we proceed on our healing journey. And the work to be done? It's increasing our knowledge of our sexuality and how we react sexually.

It's important to keep in mind, too, that all the work we do continues. In a sense, we've embarked on a never-ending journey of self-discovery and growth. The process of examining ourselves, learning, reviewing, and growing continues. As we do this, we build and strengthen our character. We learn to act in the world with greater and greater integrity.

Understanding the Role of Sexual Fantasy

Once we understand how our response cycle works, we can move on to explore the role fantasy can play in our sexual lives. Fantasy allows us to escape from the frustrations and limits of our everyday lives. Through fantasy, a person can transform the real world into whatever he or she likes, no matter how briefly or improbably. Although it is only a make-believe excursion of the mind, fantasy can help people find excitement, adventure, self-confidence, and pleasure.

From childhood on, most people have sexual fantasies that serve a variety of functions and elicit a broad range of reactions, some pleasant or exhilarating, and others embarrassing or puzzling. At times, it can be difficult to distinguish sexual fantasy from sexual desire. Just as our awareness of hunger and thinking about what kind of food we'd like to eat can blend together, our sexual appetite may merge with thoughts about how sexual satisfaction may be obtained. Although a fantasy may be valued strictly as a piece of fiction as opposed to a preview of an expected reality, this distinction does not always hold. In some cases, sexual fantasy expresses sexual desire, while in others, it *provokes* sexual desire that does not necessarily require the fantasized act for fulfillment.

Sexual fantasies range widely. Some people have fantasies about being the innocent person who is seduced by a more worldly and older partner or, in turn, being the corrupter of naive youth. Some are excited at the thought of multiple partners, of homosexual contact (a fairly common fantasy among heterosexual women and men), of wanting to be dominated (or to dominate) during the sex act, of making love in an idyllic setting, of watching others have sex, of switching partners, or of having sex with tabooed authorities, such as teachers, religious leaders, judges, or doctors. Whatever other meanings these fantasies have, they are often attempts to work through early prohibitions. Playful fantasy is a way of thumbing our noses at the forces of suppression and declaring our independence.

Just as children exercise both their curiosity and creativity when they pretend, people's sexual fantasies also draw on these elements. The desire to know about something not yet experienced, forbidden, or seemingly unattainable is often a key feature of sexual fantasies. For instance, a married woman who has always been faithful to her husband may fantasize about an extramarital liaison, or a teenage boy may fantasize about making love to a woman pictured in a *Penthouse* centerfold. In both examples, the fantasy does not necessarily mean that the person wants to actually participate in the fantasized behavior.

Functions of Sexual Fantasy[1]

Fantasies function at many different levels to boost our self-confidence, provide a safety valve for pent-up feelings, or increase sexual excitement. They may also let us triumph over the forces that prove troublesome in our everyday world.

Fantasy and sexual desire often merge. People with low levels of sexual desire typically have few sexual fantasies and often benefit from treatment that helps them form positive fantasies. Many times, sexual fantasies are used to induce or enhance sexual arousal; and, while fantasies are often combined with masturbation to provide a source of turn-on when a partner is not available, fantasies are also extremely common during sexual activity with someone else.

For some, the use of fantasy provides an initial boost to getting things underway. Others use fantasy to move from a leisurely, low-key sexual level into a more passionate state. Sexual fantasies can also enhance both the psychological and physiological parts of sexual response in many ways. They can counteract boredom, focus thoughts and feelings (to help avoid distractions or pressures), boost our self-image (in our fantasies, we can assume our desired physical attributes and need not worry about breast or penis size or body weight), and provide us with an ideal partner (or partners) who suit all our needs.

Sexual fantasies can also provide a safe, protected environment for engaging the imagination and letting our sexual feelings roam. They are safe because they are private and fictional: Privacy ensures that fantasies are undiscoverable, while the fictional makeup of our fantasies relieves us of personal accountability.

Another safety feature of fantasies lies in having control to the point of being able to end the fantasy abruptly if it becomes uncomfortable or threatening. Without such safety, the erotic value of most people's fantasies would probably decrease substantially.

Sexual fantasy can immensely enlarge our erotic repertoire. It helps us tap into our personal releasers for passion; and, when part of a full, sexual relationship, it's not at all a sign of frustrated or immature sexuality. Numerous books have appeared in recent years popularizing fantasy as a normal feature of our erotic lives, and they have provided much needed license, particularly for women, to enjoy fuller sexual expression.[2]

It is important to consider the issue of whether our sexual fantasies should be kept secret or shared with our partner. Feelings that remain secret often center on anxieties about certain sexual practices (for example, "I'm uncomfortable telling my partner that I like to have my nipples stimulated during sex because she'll think I'm unmanly.") or dissatisfaction with aspects of a partner's sexual approach or behavior (for example, "I feel neglected when my partner goes to sleep shortly after he reaches orgasm."). In such cases, communicating our feelings can help dispel frustrations and increase sexual satisfaction.

We all need to preserve some islands of privacy, but we also need to take some risks to let our lover in on what turns us on. Many times, we'll find that our partner will agree. Even if our partner doesn't share our particular erotic inclinations, he or she may open up and share his or her fantasies. Sharing fantasies opens up possibilities of greater intimacy and more leeway for experimentation.

Sex therapist Joseph Nowinski, in his book *Men, Love, & Sex*, distinguishes between using fantasies as the main method of getting sexually excited and using them as one of several techniques. He says, "If you should find yourself in a relationship in which you have to rely on fantasy as your main method of getting sexually aroused, you might need to assess that relationship to discover why it is that other sources of arousal are closed off to you. On the other hand, if you simply use fantasy as one of several ways of getting turned on, you need not be concerned about it."[3]

It may be difficult at first to share fantasies with your partner, so try talking first about erotic movies or literature that turns you on. You might also look through some magazines for pictures and comment on what images and associations appeal to you. The more you can tune into one another's specific releasers of passion through detailed fantasy, the more your lovemaking will become filled with fresh adventure.

You may find it hard to tolerate your partner's fantasy life because you wonder why the real you isn't good enough to satisfy your partner. It's as if you have a silent competitor against whom you can never measure up. This line of thinking is founded on the faulty premise that you are responsible for turning your partner on. It also fails to recognize that everyone has a secret fantasy life that is larger than one's lover, and your partner's enjoyment of fantasy need not mean you are inadequate. Your partner's bringing a personal fantasy into your relationship for the first time can mean that you are all the more special. While the content of the fantasy may not have to do with you, the act of sharing surely does.

Another important dimension of fantasy is the extent to which it is acted out. The important issue is to find the right meeting point between the illusion or fantasy and the real world. You may prefer not to enact a particular fantasy with your partner, or you may prefer to play out only a part of it. Limits need to be set, and one of them may be that the play remains contained within the privacy of the couple. Intimacy depends on such limits.

A Word of Caution for Sexual Anorexics and Sex Addicts

For many sexual anorexics and sex addicts, fantasy was often part of the obsession and, hence, part of the problem: fantasies focused on the pursuit of the unreal. They supported destructive, dangerous, or high-risk sex, or terrifying fears of the consequences of being sexual. In talking about sexual fantasy, this chapter is NOT promoting a return to old obsessions; *the goal for both sexual anorexics and sex addicts is, instead, to leave obsessional life behind.*

The suggestions and guidelines offered in this chapter are all designed to help create fantasies that support healthy sexuality—positive fantasies that can help sexual anorexics or sex addicts reclaim their sexual vitality without putting themselves in jeopardy. Used in this way, fantasy becomes an extremely powerful tool for *affirming* sexuality.

Therapists working with sexual anorexics and sex addicts often recommend creating "a sex plan." Just as someone struggling with an eating disorder learns to make a food plan, so can we all create a sex plan.

A sex plan contains three components, the first of which is a list of activities we no longer wish to do. A sex addict, for example, might include no longer having sex with prostitutes, and a sexual anorexic might include no longer avoiding intimate settings.

The second component is to establish boundaries—a list of places or situations we will avoid because they don't help our recovery or spiritual growth. An alcoholic who used to regularly drink in bars, for example, will decide to avoid bars. A sex addict who frequented massage parlors looking for prostitutes will avoid the parts of town in which these establishments are located. Sexual anorexics will avoid the distancing strategies that are part of their aversion cycle. Whereas sex addicts would rule out activities that used to bring trouble, sexual anorexics will rule out those things that kept them "safe." They will, for example, stop staying up later than their partner—which they commonly did to ensure that their partner would be asleep and thus unavailable for sex. The goal here is to avoid putting one's self in jeopardy. It's a way to avoid risk.

The third component involves choosing specific goals toward which we will work. What is healthy sexuality for us? To answer this question, both sexual anorexics and sex addicts must first define what they don't want. For the former, this means identifying exactly what terrifies them, and for the latter, identifying what got them into trouble.

Here is where healthy fantasy enters the picture. Fantasy becomes a way for us to articulate what our sex plan is all about. We imagine (or fantasize, if you will) what we want and are working toward. Fantasy becomes a way to articulate our goals as sexual beings. Visualizing ourselves in healthy and rewarding sexual situations helps to lift us out of a life lived at the extremes and to restore balance. And again, as you develop your plan and begin to use fantasy to build healthy sexuality, check in regularly with your fair witnesses for help and guidance.

Fantasy and the Sexual Response Cycle

One way to approach fantasy or imagery is to develop fantasies that can help each phase of the sexual response cycle. Below you will find a list of fantasy considerations for each phase of the response cycle, as well as issues or concerns that you should take into account in your planning. Figure 11.2 summarizes these considerations and issues.

You might refer to any of the following resources for additional information on creating sexual fantasies.

- *Intimate Play: Creating Romance in Everyday Life* by William Betcher
- *The Sexual Healing Journey: A Guide for Survivors of Sexual Abuse* by Wendy Maltz
- *Hot Monogamy: Essential Steps to More Passionate, Intimate Lovemaking* by Patricia Love and Jo Robinson
- *Joyous Sexuality: Healing from the Effects of Family Sexual Dysfunction* by Mic Hunter
- *Discovering Sexuality That Will Satisfy You Both: When Couples Want Differing Amounts and Different Kinds of Sex* by Anne S. Hastings
- *Awakening Your Sexuality: A Guide for Recovering Women* by Stephanie Covington
- *Erotic Mind: Unlocking the Inner Sources of Sexual Passion and Fulfillment* by Jack Morin

Figure 11.2

Preparation of New Sexual Imagery

Stage of Response Cycle	Fantasy Considerations	Therapeutic Issues
1. Excitement	1. Conditions or settings of fantasy 2. New or unfamiliar activities 3. Design of new rituals 4. Body points susceptible to arousal 5. Story line of fantasy 6. Play and components of arousal 7. Initiations	1. Arranging support, contract and consultation. 2. Developing model of "healthy" fantasy. 3. Making connections with larger issues in family origin and relationship. 4. Contracting about negative or unacceptable imaging. 5. Exploring "risk" issues. 6. Permission for progress vs. perfection. 7. Task: seeking permission to fantasize.
2. Plateau	1. "Conserving" the experience 2. Breathing 3. Verbal expression 4. Playful preservation of arousal 5. Uses of the senses 6. Symbols of the moment	1. Affirmation of personal value (you deserve this). 2. Trusting self, body, partner. 3. Exploring fears — real, unreal. 4. Passion as a form of vulnerability — being known (a new form of risk). 5. What happens if I do get my needs met? 6. Boredom — and is this all there is?
3. Orgasm	1. "Functional" fantasy 2. Positions for orgasm 3. Safety 4. Payoffs of orgasm	1. What family rules am I breaking with pleasure? 2. La petite mort — loss of self. 3. Is it okay to be fully myself? 4. Letting go — and passion — as an act of trust.
4. Resolution	1. Time for sexual recovery 2. Role of touch 3. Feeling goals	1. Fear of staying connected. 2. "Tests" of sexual health — feelings afterward. 3. Spirituality and meaning. 4. The senses as gateways to higher answers.

- *The Lover Within: Opening to Energy in Sexual Practice* by Julie Henderson
- *The Art of Sexual Ecstasy: The Path of Sacred Sexuality for Western Lovers* by Margo Anand

FANTASY FOR THE AROUSAL PHASE:

- Deciding on the conditions or settings for fantasy. You may need to seek the support of your fair witnesses to be able to fantasize and to ensure that the fantasies you create are healthy.

- Thinking of activities that are new or unfamiliar. It's important to develop a model of a healthy fantasy. If orgasm only works for you if you're being hurt, you need to find an alternative.

- Creating new rituals—and imagining those rituals working. Pay attention to the fantasies you create—some may connect you to larger family-of-origin and relationship issues. Francine, for example, found she had to consider and deal with both her relationship with her father and her early masturbation experiences.

- Imagining around body points that you know are suscepti- ble to arousal. It's fine to let your imagination go, but keep in mind that it's important to be careful about images that are negative or otherwise unsupportive of your goals for healthy sexuality.

- Creating a story line of the fantasy. The story line is what happens between you and your partner. Part of what creates excitement is risk. It's important to explore what risks you're willing to take, remembering that risk can be fun, but that some risks are just plain dangerous. Pay attention to this.

- Deciding on the play components of arousal. In other words, what kind of fun can you have with this? Remember, you're looking for progress, not perfection. You're only trying to create some new imagery that will be arousing. The goal is to have fun, so be playful. Don't try too hard.

- Deciding on what would initiate your fantasy. The basic task in the excitement and arousal phase is, of course, giving yourself permission to fantasize—something closely connected to giving yourself permission to be a sexual being.

FANTASY FOR THE PLATEAU PHASE:

- Deciding what you can imagine that could conserve or prolong the plateau experience. In the plateau stage, the issues involve self-knowledge and exploration. First, it's important to affirm the personal value of all this. If you're in the plateau phase, you do deserve this pleasure, and it's fine for you to have it.

- Seeing yourself stopping to breathe. The purpose here is so you can better concentrate on and really experience your body as you go through this phase. Be in the moment! For this to work, you must trust yourself, your body, and your partner. Francine's difficulties arose at this point.

- Imagining yourself talking, expressing yourself. Imagine what you would say to your partner. If you feel uncomfortable talking during sex, you may need to explore any fears (real or unfounded) that arise during this stage.

- Thinking of playful activities that would preserve the arousal. Feelings of passion and excitement can, of course, sustain the plateau. As you think about such activities, remember that experiencing passion requires us to be open, and thus to be vulnerable. Opening to passion also requires us to take a risk—to be open and vulnerable enough to let go, particularly in such an intimate situation.

- Imagining ways to involve all the senses.

- Imagining and creating "symbols of the moment." Creating symbols will make this special time of extended pleasure preceding orgasm even more special.

FANTASY FOR THE ORGASM PHASE:

- Creating a functional fantasy. In other words, your fantasy needs to be one that you can become orgasmic with. If your fantasy doesn't have an impact, why have it! Reaching orgasm creates profound pleasure. Many of us, however, grew up with rules against feeling pleasure. Fantasy is an excellent way to "act as if" you're experiencing pleasure you thought was forbidden you.

- Imagining various positions for orgasm. Numerous books depicting a variety of intercourse positions are available at most bookstores. The *Kamasutra* is one of the most ancient and well known, depicting literally hundreds of intercourse positions; various editions are available.

- Imagining and creating trust. For orgasm to work, both partners need to feel safe and trusted because orgasm basically requires letting go and diving into passion. It's a profound act of trust. The French have a phrase for orgasm, *la petite mort*, which means "the little death." In a sense, orgasm is about the loss of self. A little bit of me "dies" in order to do this with you. Can we turn ourselves over to this peak experience in which we "die" a little in order to reach the peak? Is it okay to be fully ourselves? Will our bodies carry us through this? If we allow passion to overtake us, will we be safe? We have to ask ourselves whether this is all acceptable.

- Thinking about the payoffs of the orgasm. The payoffs are over and above the mere pleasure of orgasm. What do I want to happen when I have this orgasm? What do I want to occur between me and this other person?

FANTASY FOR THE RESOLUTION PHASE:

- Fantasizing and imagining enough time to enjoy the beauty of the sexual recovery period. Imagine and create a window of time to truly be part of that.

- Imagining the role of touch. Touch is a way to stay connected with your partner. In the resolution stage, a fear of staying connected can arise. This may seem illogical, but many people have had bad experiences with sex and in relationships; their fear of connection is valid. One good test of the healthiness of sex is to examine our feelings afterwards. If we feel good, we can be fairly certain we're in the healthy range. If we have immediate remorse and feelings shut down, we need to talk with our fair witnesses for help and feedback.

- Thinking how you want to feel at this point. In other words, think about what would feel good for you now during this stage. It's in this stage, too, that people experience realizations about spirituality and meaning. "This person means a lot to me, and it's remarkable that we are able to do this together," for example. Here we can receive some obvious reinforcement that the senses can be gateways to higher awareness.

KEY QUESTIONS

In workshops and in my counseling experience, the following questions are often asked when we talk about sexual knowledge.

What do I really need to know? I mean, sometimes I feel disappointed, like "Is this all there is?"
Regardless of what we know about sex, there's always more we can learn. Having a feeling of "Is this all there is?" indicates that we need to know more. And the more we learn, the more rewarding sex can be. Become your own expert!

Do we really know anything about sex?
Yes, of course, we do. To imply that we don't know much about sex and can't learn more flies in the face of much research and the experience of countless people who have worked to improve their sex lives with very gratifying results. Learning more about sex can make a dramatic—and wonderful—difference in our lives.

Is anyone ever really sexually satisfied?
This question can only be asked from an obsessional point of view. Hidden within this question is the disbelief that sex can be a daily, regular part of our lives and that we can feel good about it.

ISSUES

Many sexual anorexics struggle with the following issues in reference to sexual knowledge. Some of these issues have been explored at greater length in this or previous chapters; for those which have not, a brief discussion is included here. Read the issues carefully, noting the ones that apply to you. Then use those issues as discussion points with your partner and/or fair witnesses.

✾ Having no preparation or knowledge to prepare for life as a sexual person.

This is true for many, many Americans, and it's a huge problem. We have no good way to communicate either the mechanics or values of sexuality. I do believe it's the province of the parents to communicate values about sexuality. However, many parents are also remarkably ill-equipped to talk knowledgeably about sex. Many children and young adults are stumbling about in this area just as did their parents and grandparents. Information is available (refer to the recommended resources at the end of this book). Seek it out. Learn. You'll be very happy you did.

✾ Realizing obsession prevented knowing basic sex information.

An obsessive preoccupation can get us stuck in a bad situation, and prevent us from getting ourselves out. Information reduces the power of obsession just as it's the key to a different life.

✾ Perceiving life as separate and unrelated to sexual issues.

It's simply impossible to separate our sexuality from the rest of our lives. At a retreat I attended for a monastic order, sexual issues arose many times. It's impossible to deny one's sexual nature.

✾ Discovering that bad information was simply confirmed by cycles of shame and dysfunction.

This problem often begins early in life when a child is given inaccurate or inappropriate sexual messages. The child goes on to have one or more bad experiences related to this information, concludes that the information has been confirmed (often by cycles of shame and dysfunction), and carries the attitude well into adulthood. Once this person discovers the error, however, he or she is well on the road to change and recovery.

❊ Operating on the basis of rules versus information.

Most families give their children many rules about sex, but little information. Sometimes these rules are based on accurate information and are basically appropriate. More often, however, the rules are not helpful, or are disregarded by the adults. In the latter case, kids eventually discover the double standard, which creates internal conflicts for them as they try to make sense of the disparity between their parents' rules and behaviors. If your rules said that sex was bad, rather than inevitable, important, and very much worth being informed about, those rules did you a disservice.

❊ Living in denial precludes any need to learn more about sex.

Living in denial precludes any opportunity to learn, change, and grow. Denial will only make our difficulties worse.

TASKS

The list on the following pages contains twenty statements about sex. Some are true, others false. Fill in your answers (or do this with your partner and write your answers on a separate sheet or in your journal).

The purpose of this exercise is only to show how much there is to know about human sexuality, and that all of us can benefit from learning more. There's no passing or failing grade here! Just keep in mind that by learning more, your sexual experiences will be more fun and fulfilling for you *and* your partner!

TWENTY FACTS ABOUT SEX QUIZ[4]

1. ____ The larger a man's penis, the more pleasurable sex will be for his partner.

2. ____ Sexual fantasies are common for both women and men.

3. ____ Oral sex is simply not something a normal, well-mannered woman would engage in.

4. ____ People over age forty or fifty can find sex more pleasurable than when they were in their twenties or thirties.

5. ____ The most common and effective way women can reach orgasm is through vaginal penetration by the man's penis during intercourse.

6. ____ The closer and more interdependent a couple are, the greater their sexual satisfaction.

7. ____ A rush to intercourse and orgasm for men leaves many women feeling unloved and unsatisfied.

8. ____ Trying new places and times for lovemaking can help keep sex exciting in a long-term relationship.

9. ____ If, while making love, a man can't have an erection, there's no way his partner will feel satisfied with their lovemaking.

10. ____ Time of day, location, energy levels of each partner, and their sense of well-being all play a critical role in sexual satisfaction.

II. ____ When it comes to sex, women are just as concerned about performance as men.

12. ____ Women tend to be more spontaneous in lovemaking than men.

13. ____ The "missionary position" for intercourse (female on her back with male on top) offers great potential for variety, and many men and women find it extremely satisfying.

14. ____ For the man, a slow, unhurried attitude will help make his **female** partner feel more relaxed and more open to the physical intimacy.

15. ____ Sex researchers have found that 75 percent of men reach orgasm within two minutes of starting intercourse.

16. ____ Masturbation is both physically and emotionally harmful.

17. ____ Having a hysterectomy means the end of sexual activity.

18. ____ Sharing our sexual secrets with a partner can enhance the relationship because we often feel an exaggerated sense of shame about this aspect of our sexuality.

19. ____ When used in conjunction with other forms of stimulation (touching, stroking, kissing), fantasy is very effective in enhancing sexual excitement and pleasure.

20. ____ Many postmenopausal women experience an ebb in sexual desire, but the causes may be more than just physical.

ANSWERS:

1. False. Study after study shows that there is simply no evidence that penis size correlates with sexual satisfaction. Rather than becoming fixated on penis size, it's much more useful to develop loving intimacy with your partner, no matter what your "equipment" size.

2. True. As recently as the 1970s, women's sexual fantasies were taken to be a sign of illness. A healthy, sexually active married woman simply did not entertain sexual fantasies. Since then, we've learned that sexual fantasies are very common, both for men and women.

3. False. Concerns about oral sex can be traced to cultural or behavioral myths. It is neither dirty nor degrading in loving relationships. One major study of married women showed that 87 percent of the respondents performed oral sex on their partner. Other studies have shown that many women rated cunnilingus, or oral stimulation of the clitoris, as their most satisfying sexual activity.

4. True. As we age, more experience with sex and greater comfort with (and knowledge about) our bodies enable men and women to achieve greater sexual satisfaction for themselves and their partner.

5. False. While the penis is the male organ most sensitive to stimulation, the clitoris, rather than the vagina, is the most sensitive in women. The direct stimulation of the clitoris, either manually or by the tongue, is more likely to elicit a woman's orgasm.

6. True. It is the honesty, intimacy, and mutual respect present in a healthy, loving relationship that create deep sexual satisfaction.

7. True. Women often view foreplay differently than men, who see it only as a prelude to something grander—

longer time during foreplay to become aroused and orgasmic. (Also refer to question 11.)

8. True. Women in particular often complain about the rigid, mechanical patterns of lovemaking by their partners. Trying new places and times for lovemaking can help keep sex exciting in a long-term relationship. A getaway weekend, or even a surprise evening away from home in a hotel, can pump enthusiasm into life's routines. Try new lovemaking positions and activities too.

9. False. Even when a man cannot maintain an erection regularly, there are still lots of ways he can provide his partner with pleasure. Oral sex, use of a vibrator, and manual stimulation are all options. Creativity and flexibility are vital.

10. True. Being exhausted, uncomfortable, stressed, worried, or preoccupied with a concern will all distract from sexual pleasure. Time of day, location, energy levels of each partner, and their sense of well-being all play a critical role in sexual satisfaction.

11. False. Women are much less performance oriented than men. Sex for women is a process of shared contact and communication rather than a mad scramble to achieve certain goals.

12. True. See answers to questions 7, 8, and 11.

13. True. Though some claim this position is too traditional and ordinary, so many men and women find it extremely satisfying that it is the most common position practiced by most couples. It is not, however, considered the ideal position for women who would like to climax during intercourse but have difficulty doing so. It is easier for a woman to reach orgasm when she is on top of the man and better able to position herself to receive maximum stimulation.

14. True. Refer to answers to questions 7 and 11.

15. True.

16. False. Most sexologists now agree that masturbation is neither physically nor emotionally harmful. Many say that the pleasure, physical movement, and stress reduction gained from masturbation offer health benefits. For individuals who have lost their partner through divorce, serious illness, or death, self-stimulation can be a practical and pleasurable way of dealing with normal sexual desire.

17. False. A hysterectomy does not end sexual activity. It should have no effect at all on a woman's ability to satisfy her partner sexually, and most women continue to experience high levels of sexual desire and pleasure. Nevertheless, studies report that as many as one-third of all women who have a hysterectomy suffer from depression and loss of sexual desire for weeks or months afterwards.

18. True. Refer to information on fantasy in this chapter.

19. True. Refer to information on fantasy in this chapter.

20. True. Many postmenopausal women experience an ebb in sexual desire. This is because a woman's natural levels of the hormone estrogen decrease dramatically after menopause. Lack of sexual desire can have other causes. Some women may find they are bored with their partner's lovemaking. Many women's lives are very busy, and they are susceptible to types of stress that have traditionally inhibited male sexual desire. Anxiety over finances, business, and job stress can all impede sexual desire. Long-term loss of sexual desire may mean, too, that there are deep-seated problems in a relationship.

THE TOP TEN LIST

The following is a list of the ten most common questions men and women, respectively, ask about sex. Questions like these have long been on the minds of men and women, but today they are being asked with a new urgency. They are taken from the newsletter *Sex over 40*. (See the list of resources at the end of this book for more information on this newsletter.) Use these questions as food for thought and as a guide for your work in increasing your knowledge about human sexuality.

THE TEN MOST COMMON QUESTIONS MEN ASK ABOUT SEX

1. What do women want from men in a lovemaking relationship?
2. How can I best excite my partner?
3. What is a woman's experience of an orgasm like?
4. How should I react when my partner isn't interested in sex?
5. How can I keep sex exciting in a long-term relationship?
6. Is it common to fantasize about one person while making love to another?
7. Is masturbation beneficial or harmful?
8. How important is it to delay ejaculation?
9. Does penis size make a difference in providing sexual gratification?
10. Do men experience a drop-off in sexual desire as they age?

THE TEN MOST COMMON QUESTIONS WOMEN ASK ABOUT SEX

1. I frequently have sexual fantasies. Is this common, and what should I do about them?
2. My husband and I have a good sex life, but I still feel like masturbating. What are the benefits of masturbating and is it normal as we grow older?
3. I've never performed oral sex for my partner. How can I overcome my inhibition to give him this pleasure?
4. My partner and I have made love in the same position for many years. How can we get more variety into our lovemaking?
5. Because my husband doesn't always get an erection, he is sometimes reluctant to make love. How can I make him realize there are other ways of giving me pleasure?

6. What are the optimal conditions for good sex?
7. I can't seem to have an orgasm during intercourse. I'm not sure what the cause is, but I suspect that it may be that my husband just doesn't last long enough for me to be satisfied.
8. I'm menopausal, and I seem to have lost interest in sex. I wish I could be more excited about it. What can I do?
9. My husband no longer seems very interested in sex, but it still means a lot to me. How can I interest him?
10. My doctor has informed me that I may need a hysterectomy. I really enjoy sex now with my partner. What will be the impact of this surgery on our sex life?

YOUR SEXUAL RESPONSE CYCLE

This chapter introduced you to the human sexual response cycle. You learned how this cycle varies from person to person, as well as from time to time, for a given individual. Think about two times you've been sexual. In your journal, draw your own sexual response cycle for each occasion. When you've finished, write down the feelings you've had during each of the four phases.

A HEALTHY FANTASY

Referring to the previous exercise, now create a healthy fantasy that would enhance your pleasure during sex. Write your fantasy in your journal.

PLANNING

Together with your partner, decide on some aspects of sexuality you'd like to learn more about and/or what new activities you'd like to add to your sex life together. Make a list of them.

Next choose one or two items you'd like to work on first. Decide what you'll need to learn and/or prepare, and where you'll find the resources to do so.

Finally, set an approximate time limit for information gathering, and then give yourselves two or three weeks (or whatever feels comfortable) to try these new activities.

When you're comfortable with them and interested in again learning and/or trying something new, choose one or two more items from your list.

Move at a pace that is comfortable for *both* of you.

And remember, you can add to your list, too, as new ideas come to you!! If you're not careful, you might be working from this list for many, many years!

IN YOUR JOURNAL

Start each morning by writing your "daily pages." In addition, since this chapter focuses on sexual knowledge, include thoughts about this topic in your journal.

A CLOSING EXERCISE

✐ The closing exercise asks you and your partner to evaluate yourselves and one another. Remember, this exercise offers a wonderful opportunity for you to discover your strengths and weaknesses, as well as a chance for you and your partner to compare your perceptions of yourselves and one another.

In addition to filling out the rating scales, it will be helpful to do the following:

- Once you have filled out your scales, share the results with your fair witnesses.
- After your partner has finished, talk about your partner's perceptions too. They may differ from yours and/or those of your fair witnesses.
- If significant discrepancies exist, note them and then return to your fair witnesses to look into them more carefully.

As you work on these scales, try not to become defensive if the perceptions your partner or your fair witnesses have of you differ from your own perceptions of yourself. Let these differences—and the reasons for them—be a source of information for all of you.

If you are not currently in a relationship, ask one of your fair witnesses (therapist, sponsor, anorexia group member, Twelve Step support group member, or RCA group member, for example) to work through the scales with you.

Part 1: Focus on You

Consider your level of sexual knowledge. Are you satisfied with what you know? Would you like to know more? Do you need to know more? How would you rate your knowledge about sexuality?

Using a circle, rate yourself on the scale below. (1 = low skills, need much work; 10 = high skills, need no further work.)

Next, ask your partner to rate your sexual knowledge. Have your partner use a square to rate you.

1   2   3   4   5   6   7   8   9   10

Part 2: Focus on Your Partner

On this second scale, ask your partner to consider sexual knowledge as it applies to him or her. Is your partner satisfied with what he or she knows about sex? Would your partner like to know more? Does your partner need to know more? How much work does your partner need on sexual knowledge?

Have your partner use a circle to rate himself or herself.

Next, you rate your partner's sexual knowledge. Use a square to do so.

1   2   3   4   5   6   7   8   9   10

Knowledge

Nurturing—
We learn to trust and to open our lives to experience.

Sensuality—
Through our senses, we interact with the world around us
and become connected to it.

Self-Image—
We learn that we are good and lovable.

Self-Definition—
We develop a relationship with ourselves and come to trust
ourselves. We are trustworthy.

Comfort—
We learn that we can trust others.

Knowledge—
With the acceptance of ourselves and others, we seek to grow
as people.

12

RELATIONSHIPS

Genuine love is an expression of productiveness, and implies care, respect, responsibility and knowledge. It is not an 'affect' in the sense of being affected by somebody, but an active striving for the growth and happiness of the loved person, rooted in one's own capacity to love.

—Erich Fromm
Man for Himself

A CRITICAL COMPONENT of healthy sexuality is the ability to develop and maintain intimate relationships with those of the same and opposite gender. For this reason, one of the key points on which therapists focus when working with couples is the degree of comfort each has with members of the same and opposite gender. If we are, in general, unable to form healthy relationships, we'll find it next to impossible to form intimate, erotic relationships.

Being "in love" with someone doesn't automatically ensure a life of "happily ever after." If anything, the need for the whole range of relationship skills is accentuated in such a relationship. In addition, it's important to feel comfortable with people both of the same and opposite gender. Our relationships with other people will suffer if we aren't able to do so. One of the most important skills human beings can have is the ability to create a support network around them—one that comprises *both* men and women.

Adding to our challenge is the current state of flux in gender roles and relationships in many cultures. At this point in human history, we are struggling with a profound challenge: redefining the roles of men and women, as well as our relationships with one another. Many cultures across the planet still strictly limit the relationships between men and women, and friendships with those of the opposite gender are often prohibited. Pressure is mounting, however, across the planet for greater respect and equality, particularly for women.

In our society, roles and "rules" for both men and women have been under pressure to change for the better part of this century, and one of the biggest questions turns on the issue of having friends of both genders. How exactly do we do this? A friend of mine, Jack, who's about forty-five, tells a story that exemplifies this conundrum. When Jack was twenty, one of his best friends, Mike, met a young woman and eventually married her. Mike's wife, Julie, and Jack hit it off quite well and grew to be good friends. As Jack said, "It was truly platonic; I would never have dreamed of coming on to my friend's wife. Both Julie and I recognized the mutual attraction, we even talked about it. We agreed, too, that we would never be sexual. And Mike was fine with this too. We all trusted one another."

Jack's parents knew the couple, too, and as Julie's name began coming up in conversations more often, they became concerned. One day, Jack's parents confronted him. "They were both convinced that Julie and I were having an affair. No amount of argument by me could convince them that this was just a friendship. They simply didn't believe that it was possible for me or any guy to have a close relationship with a woman, married or not, and not have it be sexual. I guess it was a generational difference. I finally gave up arguing with them, and solved the problem by just never mentioning her name again."

Recent changes in what is expected of men and women—

and how we relate to one another—make efforts to form healthy relationships all the more difficult. Men and women need first to work on their same-sex relationships. These relationships are vital because without them, our ability to sustain an intimate relationship will be lessened dramatically.

We simply must create and nurture other close relationships, because without them, we have no opportunity to gain a perspective on our intimate ones. If we're only close and intimate with one person, and all the other people with whom we interact are simply casual friends, for example, we can't help but overload that one special relationship. The vitality of special or romantic relationships is affected by how well we are supported by other good, close friends in whom we can confide. It's both unfair and unrealistic to expect one person to supply all our needs. If we depend on that one person too much, we over-ask and over-invest in that relationship—to the detriment of both partners.

We can have our relationship needs met in many ways, but all require having at least a few really good friends. Unfortunately, strong obstacles confront both men and women in this task, some societal, and others grounded in family history. I have seen women, for example, who very much like being with and talking to men, but who are not the least interested in getting close to other women. There can be many reasons for this. Experiences with their mothers characterized by extreme betrayal and mistrust, for example, can lead women to transfer those attitudes to women in general. Regardless of the reason, however, when these women join a women's group, they often discover that one reason they'd been in degrading and abusive relationships with men is that they didn't know that they could get their needs met elsewhere. With this revelation, and the gift of good women friends, their self-esteem improves dramatically. In addition, they no longer miss out on the opportunity to learn more about their sexuality by being with other women.

Men face even more difficult problems in trying to develop close male friends. The recent McGill Report on male intimacy noted that men basically have a difficult time bonding in our culture. The researchers found, for example, that out of every twenty men, only *one* had more than one best friend. Think about this! The report also verified a clear link between male vulnerability to addiction and a failure to bond with other men.

In this society—and for men in particular—having same-gender friends also forces us to confront the issue of homophobia, a fear of people of the same gender. This subject could itself fill a book, but suffice it to say that there's not a man alive in this country—gay or straight—who didn't at some time live with the fear of being called a homosexual. These negative and prejudicial attitudes often interfere with men's ability and willingness to get emotionally close to one another.

Our culture injures men and women differently, as writer Helen Block Lewis pointed out so well some years ago in her book *Psychic War in Men and Women*.

Men as "Expendable Warriors"

Lewis refers to men as "expendable warriors" who are taught to avoid emotional attachment to others. Modern-day warriors don't fight so much as they compete, and this culture is rife with competition. In the business environment, for example, literally everyone is a competitor, both people from other companies as well as one's co-workers. We never know who might be after our job, or when our boss will fire us. We're expendable. Given such perceptions and work environment, we may find it illogical to build true friendships. Men also feel a pressure to compete in many other areas of their lives, including wealth acquisition, sports prowess, and the attractiveness of their mates.

For many men in this culture, self-worth is closely bound up in what they do and provide. They see their role as providers for their spouses and families, and the more they can provide, the better men they are. Consequently, when men lose their jobs, the effect is particularly devastating. Women invest less emotionally in their work; self-worth for women also comes through close friends and family members. Not so for men—remember the McGill Report?!

Does this scenario sound a bit familiar? Dad comes down to breakfast, and the family is getting ready for the day, bustling around, chatting, and suddenly he realizes that no one has talked to *him* in the last twenty minutes. He wonders to himself, "If the checks just kept coming, would they even notice whether I was here or not?" Men learn that they are only as good as what they do or bring in for the family; who they are as a person is not so important, so why invest emotionally in others?

This curriculum for men is powerful and ubiquitous. I remember, for example, when I was just a junior in high school and dating a young woman with whom I was very enamored. When I went to pick her up for dates, I'd drive over in my family's 1950 Chevrolet, an old farm car literally held together with baling wire. My chief competitor for her attention was a guy whose father ran a Chevy dealership in town. "Tom" would always show up in a new Impala convertible or Corvette, and, of course, the contrast was not lost on anyone involved! While I think this young woman genuinely liked me, she *was* impressed with the other guy's car and the appearance it made. What men learn from this curriculum, then, is that we're only as good as what we can do or can produce. Who we are as a human being is not of particular importance.

Women as "Inferior Child Bearers"

Women, too, are caught up in this system. Let's look at diamond engagement rings. When a woman receives one—and, of course, it's the man who gives the ring to her, she doesn't buy it herself—what does she do? She immediately shows it to every other woman she knows, and the bigger the ring is—in other words, the more money her fiancé has spent—the bigger the sighs and raves. What message does this give to men?

In a competitive and exploitive culture such as ours, women, whom Lewis calls the "inferior child bearers," are injured through discounting of ability and denial of leadership. The arguments should be familiar: Women can't lead because they're too emotional, because they need to take care of kids, because the Bible says their place is in the home, because they aren't tough enough, because they become irrational and unreliable at "certain times"(!) every month. Women struggle, because of oppression, with power and victimization issues.

Under the influence of addiction, men in this culture tend to be excessive in behaviors that objectify their partners and require little emotional involvement (practicing voyeuristic, anonymous, and/or exploitive sex). Women who are addicted, however, choose forms of excessive behavior that distort power by either gaining control over others or being a victim (practicing fantasy sex, seduction, and trading sex). Women sex addicts use sex for power, for control, and for attention.

In such a system, men become human "doings" rather than human "beings." This situation angers many women, of course, because they want men to be personal, gentle, loving, involved, and emotional, yet women participate in perpetuating the very system that creates the kind of men they don't like. And men? They're caught in a series of wicked double binds.

A corollary in the "expendable warrior" curriculum of "avoid attachment" teaches men to protect themselves against loss. Men in our culture are asked to take all the initiative. It's their responsibility to ask women for dates, to ask them to dance, to propose marriage, to be "in charge" of the household and the marriage, and so on. Women, taking the opposite role, are responsible for waiting for men to do their part. (This is the point of origin for much of women's efforts to "manipulate" men to get what they want. The curriculum teaches women that it's not okay to be assertive and ask for what they want, so they resort to the backdoor of manipulation.)

Eventually, men learn to remain detached and to objectify others, particularly women. Following this logic, it makes good sense to turn women into sex objects because it's easier to be rejected by an object than by a human being with whom you are connected and vulnerable. This objectification, combined with a belief that they have to initiate all activity, is precisely how we make men into rapists and women into victims. Combine lessons in detachment and objectification with the idea that they are only as good as their money or their job, and it should be no surprise that men don't have the relationship-oriented skills they or the women in their lives would like them to have.

In many Native American and other cultures in which women have respected positions, in which roles of both genders are equally respected, in which decision-making and leadership roles are balanced between genders, much of the pathology discussed in this book—rape, child abuse, prostitution—is seldom present. This is why moving to a point where both genders enjoy similar respect and have similar opportunities is of incredible importance.

In this culture, men and women have long been, in a sense, living in separate camps, and as a result have had little opportunity to relate with and know one another as people, without the involvement of sexuality. This situation only serves to perpetuate misinformation and misperceptions; hence, the enormous importance of establishing genuine cross-gender friendships that aren't somehow eroticized, as well as good same-gender relationships. Such relationships supply important information and break down stereotypes—all critical to having a healthy sexual relationship.

Watching my son, David, growing up let me see that these old patterns may be finally changing for the better. During high school, my son spent a lot of his time with a group of four girls and three guys, all very good friends, and *only* good friends. They did not date within the group. It was not unusual to find them all crashed on our living-room floor, though we never worried about this because it was clear that they weren't interested in being sexual with one another. They did, of course, date other people, which was often a source of endless conversations when "the pack," as I called them, were together. Who was dating whom, how it went, how attached they were, and so on. They received a lot of feedback from one another, and the group provided them, I think, a lot of comfort.

One day, David came home from school and said to me, "You know, Dad, women are very strange." And I said, "Oh, and how so?"

"Well," he replied, "the girls in the group sat all us boys down yesterday and explained to us that all of them were having their periods this week and they wanted us to go away until Friday."

Now when I was growing up, to have a discussion with a girl about her period would have just . . . well, it would simply have never happened. I'm not sure I even really knew what menstruation was when I was his age! I was astounded that these kids were able to talk about menstruation, and impressed that the young women knew and could articulate what they needed at that moment. To have a level of comfort among themselves and with the boys that let them talk about this subject is a very positive sign. It's the kind of openness within and between genders that sets the foundation for healthy sexual relationships.

Issues for Gays and Lesbians

Being gay or lesbian presents an additional dimension to efforts to form healthy same-gender and opposite-gender relationships. Gays and lesbians must not only work through the general cultural issues surrounding sexuality, but also they must face a separate set of issues regarding sexual attraction toward the same gender. In addition, they must deal with the tremendous shame and guilt over having sexual feelings for people of the same gender, and the often virulent homophobic attitudes of the straight community. Stephen's story below illustrates some of the issues gays and lesbians encounter.

Though I grew up in a very loving family, I still had very low self-esteem and a lot of self-loathing— primarily because of a congenital neurological disorder which left my arm bent. This wasn't much of a problem until I went to school. There, the other boys made fun of me constantly, beating me up, mocking my arm, and calling me faggot.

In grade school, girls became my saviors. Not only didn't they make fun of me, they protected me from the boys who were always after me. That protection was not only physical, but psychological; they helped my ego by telling me that the boys were just jealous because I had so many cute girls hanging around me. As I grew older in junior and senior high school, I identified more and more with women because of the warmth, sensitivity, and emotional openness they expressed. Basically, I hated boys, though I did have a couple good male friends in junior and senior high.

I believe that both men and women have male and female aspects. Society separates us, however, saying that men should be "all male" and vice versa for women. I, and many gay men I know, have more "feminine" characteristics, which is what draws straight women to gay men—we're not very machismo. Identifying on an emotional level with straight women is much easier for a gay man than trying to identify with a straight man. I do know straight men with these "feminine" characteristics, but in my experience, such men are very rare.

Unlike my partner, I was exposed to gay culture when I was growing up in New York City. I knew what it meant to be gay, and I didn't think it was wrong to be gay—though I certainly knew it wasn't society's preferred lifestyle! Though I personally didn't have shame about being gay, I know a lot of gay men who not only grew up in settings in which they heard a message that sex was dirty, but they got an additional one that said that sex with another man was a ticket straight to hell. Eternal damnation was the price you paid for being gay. Shame about being gay is definitely a huge, huge issue for gay men. How many straight guys get thrown out of their house for having sex with a woman? All of us know a lot of gays and lesbians who have literally been tossed out onto the street when they came out to their families.

Growing up, I was comfortable having sex with either gender; in fact, I saw myself as special because of this. My sexuality with women was very respectful, because I so valued them. With men, however, it was different story. Looking back, I can see that I objectified men as a way to get back at those mean boys in my childhood. On the other hand, I was also very deprived of male relationships for the same reason. I got to a point at which the ultimate way I could be accepted by men was to be sexual with them. It was a kind of drive to conquer them—and it led to my sexual addiction.

I never really had any problem connecting with other gay men, or with straight women, either, given my history with them. I had long identified with straight women, lesbians, and gay men, and I think this is true for most gays and lesbians.

My big challenge was to learn to identify with the straight male world and to relate to straight men. When I was in AA and SAA, I only went to gay groups—and I did get recovery from that. But my true healing happened only when I could finally identify with straight men. To be accepted by them was extremely healing for me.

Some years after recovery from chemical and sex addiction, I joined a Recovering Couples Anonymous group with my partner, thus entering the straight world even further. Everyone knows the term "homophobia." Once repressed groups like gays and lesbians find comfort in a community of our own, we can have a kind of "heterophobia." It's a fear of being vulnerable in the straight world because of how we've been so hurt by the straight society. To go back out into that world and share our truths is scary. To be able to talk about our issues in an RCA group of straight couples was difficult at first, but my partner and I were very much accepted by these people, and that was also very, very healing.

Anger Rooted in Gender Prejudice

Though prejudicial and unfounded attitudes toward gays and lesbians are clearly destructive, too many people hold equally destructive, generalized opinions about members of the same and opposite gender—opinions which I describe as anger rooted in sexuality, or sexualized rage. If you're a woman, have you ever participated in a conversation with other women in which one woman related an act that an obviously "Neanderthal" male had done? Then, when she said, "It's congenital and true about all men," the rest of the group all nodded in agreement! If you're a man, have you ever spent some time with work buddies or friends commiserating about the emotionality and trauma of someone's "high-maintenance" spouse? This kind of generalization to all members of a gender is an example of sexualized rage.

A wonderful and humorous example of generalized thinking, one which I love to talk to audiences about, was depicted in a famous scene in the movie *When Harry Met Sally*. It's the scene where Sally (Meg Ryan) fakes an orgasm for Harry (Billy Crystal) in a restaurant.

The context of this scene is very instructive, so let me reconstruct it for you. While sitting with Sally in a restaurant, Harry says that *he* can always tell if a woman is really having an orgasm or merely faking it. Keep in mind that at this point, Harry and Sally are friends, but not yet lovers. Sally responds by asking, "How can you say that when you're out of the house by 3 a.m. before the andirons get cold?"—a reference to males fleeing the bed/woman after sex. In order to demonstrate just how wrong he is, Sally proceeds to pretend she's experiencing an orgasm right there at the restaurant table, halfway through their meal, and she gives a *very* convincing performance. As she's finishing, a waiter asks an older woman sitting a few tables away what she'd like to order and, glancing in Sally's direction, the woman replies, "I'll have whatever it is that *she's* having."

Clearly this is, on the surface, an hilarious scene, but notice that it's founded on an implicit anger between members of the opposite sex. Each of these characters holds a belief that says this is the way that all men—or women—are. The effect of this kind of attitude is to depersonalize and objectify our relationships with the opposite gender.

It's very important for our own happiness and for the health of all our relationships to be aware of when we do this in our own lives. Do you harbor angry feelings toward men or women? Do you make broad-brush statements that are prejudicial and angry? Pay attention to how you talk about men and women, and make the needed changes.

As a final point, when we begin to understand how our culture has mistreated both men and women, some reaction is, of course, appropriate. Writer Robert Bly describes this very well when he says that the appropriate feeling for women in our culture is anger over the way that they have been dismissed, disregarded, and disenfranchised. The appropriate feeling for men is mourning over what they have missed in their lives by not ever really knowing other men and by objectifying women.

Part of our focus must now be on deciding what we have to do to repair the damage between sexes. We all have opinions about one another, but global judgments that are inherently inaccurate only serve to diminish our own sexuality. Until we change, these attitudes will continue to subtly damage all our relationships.

KEY QUESTIONS

In workshops and in my counseling experience, the following questions are often asked when we talk about building relationships and living with a partner.

When I watch television shows like Friends *or* Relativity, *the close relationships the characters seem to have make me jealous. Do people* really *have friends like that?*
Yes, and not only is it possible, it's imperative for having healthy sexuality.

Can you be part of a community of men and women and have friendships that don't become sexual?
Yes. To have healthy sexuality, we must have a community of friends—but to do so requires us to change. We must look at ourselves to discover our deficits and inadequacies so we can improve our relationships with both men and women. We need to think and act differently. All of this

requires taking a risk—to accept that we can change and to try.

By committing to risk and change, we are, in a sense, taking a Seventh Step. In the Twelve Step tradition, Step Seven is really an act of faith. It means trusting that a Higher Power will help us with these efforts. Anyone who sets out on the path toward greater personal growth must make a leap of faith that they can succeed and that they will be okay. Without such faith, growth and change are not possible.

ISSUES

Many sexual anorexics struggle with the following issues in reference to relationships. Some of these issues have been explored at greater length in this or previous chapters; for those which have not, a brief discussion is included here. Read the issues carefully, noting the ones that apply to you. Then use those issues as discussion points with your partner and/or fair witnesses.

❋ Lacking comfort with the same sex.

❋ Lacking comfort with the opposite sex.

❋ Experiencing gender shame or embarrassment about one's own sex.

❋ Separating friendship from the erotic.

❋ Seeing sex or using sex as a weapon and means of control. It's not uncommon for people who are uncomfortable with their sexuality, or who have unresolved issues about themselves and/or those of the opposite gender, to use sex as a weapon (by withholding sex or being sexual with someone else, for example) and means of control in a struggle between genders.

✻ Using sex with other emotions such as loneliness or fear. During childhood, some people inadvertently eroticized their feelings. Here's how this can happen. If, as a child, for example, you often felt very lonely, fearful, and anxious, and your only way of coping with those feelings was to masturbate regularly, at some point your feelings become connected with feeling sexual. Eventually, you no longer experience loneliness, fear, or anxiety; instead you have only sexual feelings.

As an adult, someone who has eroticized feelings will not be able to connect with anyone without being sexual. For a sex addict to have nonsexual friends, for example, would be an exercise in futility. Why would he or she do that? Sexual anorexics who grew to adulthood with this same problem are just as eroticized, only they have a negative balance. Obsessing about *not* having sex is also a way for them to avoid their feelings of pain, loneliness, shame, and so on.

✻ Being jealous as a result of old addictive and obsessive beliefs.
"Women are unreliable and fickle." Many men have experienced this core attitude, and, as a result, they harbor feelings of distrust for women. Conversely, more than a few women distrust men, assuming that they're ready at the wink of an eye to hop into bed with another woman.

I found myself falling into this trap some years ago when I was standing in an airport check-in line behind a twenty-something couple. The woman was giving a *very* fond, tearful farewell to a man to whom she was clearly engaged. After finally saying good-bye to this guy, she got on the plane and sat in the seat in front of mine, next to a fellow who was quite handsome. She had no sooner sat down than she began engaging him in a flirtatious and seductive way. So I said to myself, "Yup, that's the way women are." But, of course, that's *not* true. I *know* this based on years of professional training and work, and from my own experience with trustworthy women.

Someplace in my head, however, this belief about the unreliability of women was still floating around.

Women must also deal with similar biases about men. Such deep-seated attitudes truly interfere with creating meaningful, fulfilling relationships with those of the opposite gender. Changing such attitudes won't happen by accident or over night, though—it requires honesty, open communication, and a willingness to look at others without the filter of our biases.

TASKS

The problem of sexualized rage, wherein a few experiences are generalized to all experiences, haunts sexual anorexics. Maintaining this rage merely serves as one more way to keep obsessions finely honed and focused. Phrases like "all men are . . ." and "all the men do . . ." signify sexualized rage. The importance of building sexual community requires us to confront these stereotypes and explore our visions of men and women. To do so, we must first notice the contrast between peers who support obsession and those who support change.

Look at the people around you. Who is supporting your efforts to change? There is no point in surrounding yourself with people who are only interested in talking about how bad men/women are. This is precisely why anyone following this program is encouraged to pull together a group of fair witnesses who can see the truth *and* who are willing to tell you— people who will support your efforts to move on to healthier, more open expressions of your sexual life.

The stories Rick, Nancy, and Alan tell below are examples of the rules and assumptions about how men and women "are" that we learn in this culture. You'll find these stories helpful in doing the exercises that follow.

RICK:

It took me a long time to see the assumptions I'd been holding about men and women. I'll just list some of them. Women are second class and submissive, and they should please a man whenever he wants pleasing. Women are there to reward men if they do a good job, and so on. Women control sex, but don't really enjoy it. Women will get men in trouble. Women are desirable, but unattainable.

Men are supposed to satisfy women. Be aggressive. Be responsible for and protect women. Men don't share their affections, and they don't cry. Other men are competitors for women, jobs, prestige, and so on, so be careful of them. Homosexuality is very bad.

NANCY:

My mother was selfless and took a lot of crap at home. The way I saw it was that women were either child-bearing, overweight, selfless wives or seductive, vampirelike maneaters. I resented the Mom role, seeing no future in being a beast of burden. The vamps got the attention and were sought after based on their looks. As long as I had to be a woman, I decided I was going to make the most of it until my looks ran out, then settle for being the beast of burden, a wife. Women were sex objects and should be beautiful and sexy to please men.

Men were the leaders—strong, powerful, calling the shots. I used men to meet my own needs, avoiding emotional entanglements, and stopping them if they wanted more in a relationship than I did. I thought that men wanted two kinds of women: women they could have sex with OR women they took to nice places and eventually married. I was in the former category. I felt men basically needed women for sex and to raise their kids and keep house. Men were the rulers, had the power, made the decisions, earned the money.

I learned that men controlled women, and that was because women couldn't make up their minds and had to be told what to do, especially sexually. I learned to read men's minds and bodies. What women wanted didn't count. I basically thought men were unfeeling and only went out with me for sex. I felt safe, however, only with women. I craved nurturing and felt I could only get this from other women; men were incapable of nurturing.

ALAN:

First, I thought I had to be exclusively straight or gay. My father was chauvinistic and condescending toward women. I learned that men don't cry or touch one another, nor do they acknowledge their feelings. Women are passive objects. I felt tremendous pressure to conform and to date women, denying my homosexuality. Other kids mocked my interests in music and drama, which were seen as feminine.

BELIEFS ABOUT MEN AND WOMEN

After looking at the examples above, create your own list of "beliefs" about men and women. List these beliefs in your journal. Make two lists, one for each gender. Then answer the following questions.

1. How comfortable do you feel with members of the same gender?

2. What do you like and dislike about them?

3. How comfortable do you feel with members of the opposite gender?

4. What do you like and dislike about them?

BELIEFS ABOUT GAYS AND LESBIANS

Think about your beliefs about gays or lesbians. List these beliefs in your journal. Again make two lists, one for each gender. Then answer the following questions.

1. How comfortable do you feel with gay men?

2. What do you like and dislike about them?

3. How comfortable do you feel with lesbian women?

4. What do you like and dislike about them?

PLANNING

Explore the results of the above work with your partner and your fair witnesses. You might also consider encouraging your partner to complete the above exercises, too, and then talk about and compare one another's results.

IN YOUR JOURNAL

Begin each morning by writing your "daily pages." In addition, since this chapter focuses on relationships, include thoughts about this topic in your journal.

A CLOSING EXERCISE

✐   The closing exercise asks you and your partner to evaluate yourselves and one another. Remember, this exercise offers a wonderful opportunity for you to discover your strengths and weaknesses, as well as a chance for you and your partner to compare your perceptions of yourselves and one another.

In addition to filling out the rating scales, it will be helpful to do the following:

- Once you have filled out your scales, share the results with your fair witnesses.
- After your partner has finished, talk about your partner's perceptions too. They may differ from yours and/or those of your fair witnesses.
- If significant discrepancies exist, note them and then return to your fair witnesses to look into them more carefully.

As you work on the scales, try not to become defensive if the perceptions your partner or your fair witnesses have of you differ from your own perceptions of yourself. Let these differences—and the reasons for them—be a source of information for all of you.

If you are not currently in a relationship, ask one of your fair witnesses (therapist, sponsor, anorexia group member, Twelve Step support group member, or RCA group member, for example) to work through the scales with you.

Part 1: Focus on You

On the first scale, consider the quality of your relationships with men and women. Do you have good friends of the same gender? Of the opposite gender? Are these relationships all that you'd like them to be? How would you rate yourself in this area?

Using a circle, rate yourself on the scale. (1 = low skills, need much work; 10 = high skills, need no further work.)

Next, ask your partner to rate you on relationships. Have your partner use a square to rate you.

I   2   3   4   5   6   7   8   9   10

Part 2: Focus on Your Partner

On this second scale, ask your partner to consider the quality of his or her relationships with men and women. Does your partner have good friends of the same gender? Of the opposite gender? Are these relationships all that your partner would like them to be? How much work does your partner need to do in the area of relationships?

Have your partner use a circle to rate himself or herself.

Next, you rate your partner on relationships. Use a square to do so.

I   2   3   4   5   6   7   8   9   10

Nurturing—
We learn to trust and to open our lives to experience.

Sensuality—
Through our senses, we interact with the world around us
and become connected to it.

Self-Image—
We learn that we are good and lovable.

Self-Definition—
We develop a relationship with ourselves and come to trust
ourselves. We are trustworthy.

Comfort—
We learn that we can trust others.

Knowledge—
With the acceptance of ourselves and others, we seek to grow
as people.

Relationships—
Based on what we have learned, we make the leap of trying to
live in new ways.

PARTNERS

When a man and woman with significant spiritual and psychological affinities encounter each other and fall in love, if they have evolved beyond the level of problems and difficulties, if they are beyond the level of merely struggling to make their relationship "work," then romantic love becomes the pathway not only to sexual and emotional happiness but also to the higher reaches of human growth. It becomes the context for a continuing encounter with the Self, through the process of interaction with another Self. Two consciousnesses, each dedicated to personal evolution, can provide an extraordinary stimulus and challenge to one another. Then ecstasy can become a way of life.

Romantic love is not a myth waiting to be discarded, but, for most of us, a discovery waiting to be born.

—Nathaniel Branden

AT SOME PLACE and time, out of the "pack" of humanity will emerge an individual who kindles in us a special feeling. We're attracted to this person emotionally, intellectually, physically, and erotically. This is the stuff of romance.

Romance is not, however, something that just comes with the human gene package. It's an idea that we created; and, when we did, it represented a profound shift in relationships. Author and cultural anthropologist Joseph Campbell, in his book *Hero with a Thousand Faces*, helps put this shift into perspective. In the twelfth century, he says, two things took place that changed the course of modern history. The first was the writing of the Magna Charta, a document—and an idea—that was the first step in Western culture's development of democratic government and affiliative culture based on gender respect and equality. This was an incredibly significant shift.

At the same time, ironically, French poets began writing about courtship. This, according to Campbell, was another very innovative idea because at that time, and for centuries before, the marriage of two people was a contract arranged by the families of the two partners. This contract was governed by complex rules that had nothing at all to do with whether the two individuals cared about one another. Partners did occasionally fall in love and get married, but the overwhelming majority of marriages were arranged unions designed to improve the economic, political, and social status of the families involved.

The introduction of choice fundamentally changed the nature of the marriage relationship because with choice comes responsibility and the possibility of romance. Romance doesn't appear when someone tells us we're going to marry. It springs from attraction and grows from the heart. It requires that we make ourselves vulnerable and take risks, which is precisely what's so exciting about falling in love—the risk that comes with it. A risk that this other person might not respond to us. A risk that if this person gets to know us, he or she might reject us. The more we reveal of ourselves, the greater the risk. If a friend leaves us, that's one thing. If someone for whom we feel great attraction and deep passion leaves, such a rejection strikes far deeper. In romantic relationships, there's simply a lot more on the line.

The importance of this innovation in relationships was demonstrated recently by the results of an interesting study in

China. Historically, all Chinese marriages were arranged. Today, however, only half are arranged; the rest are marriages of choice. This study compared the marital satisfaction of the two groups. By an overwhelming margin, the happiest people (*especially* women!) were those who had been able to choose their partners.

What truly intrigues me is this: that so many American couples begin with deep passion and romance only to report sooner or later that the romance has disappeared from their partnership. Or how often do we hear couples say that sex was great while they were courting one another, but once they married, the sex became dull and routine.

It seems as though there are about 85 million books on how to put romance back into our relationships. Well, I'd like to suggest an alternative—*The Dr. Carnes Simplistic Remedy*. Try honesty. Honesty about what you're really thinking. About what you're really feeling. When two people are dating, they regularly take big risks in terms of honesty. Everything seems so open—and that's part of the excitement and the romance. What happens to it?

When passion and sex melt away from a relationship, part of what's missing is the risk. The risk of being known, of taking chances, of showing who we are. Once a commitment has been made, many people unconsciously decide that they no longer need to continue putting themselves on the line. If you were totally honest with your partner about every thought you had for a whole day, I can guarantee that you'd have the most interesting day you've had in a long time!

Other factors come into play too. When we're falling in love, we can feel almost intoxicated; and new love is, literally, physiologically intoxicating to some degree. Michael Liebowitz, in *The Chemistry of Love*, underlines the importance to romantic attraction of the neuropeptide called phenylethylamine, or PEA. According to Liebowitz, PEA is critical to the chemistry of courtship. Its molecular structure parallels that of amphetamines and creates a high-arousal state. The mood-altering effect of PEA is immediate but short-lived, and its intense impact tapers off as the romance gets past the initial "limerance" stage to the bonding of the long-term attachment phase of love.

As an aside, it's not unusual to see some sex addicts regularly move from person to person, falling in love over and over again. For them, falling in love becomes the addiction. They're always searching for the "cosmically right" person, but as soon as the relationship hits those deeper levels of establishing meaning and commitment, they're gone. They find another person who is somehow better, and, of course, they needed only about five minutes to make this decision. He knew "instantly" that this was the woman who would make it all okay, or she knew that this was the man for whom she'd been searching all her life. These relationships, of course, are much more about conquest than love.

Most of us, not being sex addicts, find that it's not too difficult to cruise through the first stages of a relationship. It's when we finally reach a place where deeper issues of relationship, companionship, conflict, and differences must be confronted that we have trouble. I have always loved Scott Peck's comment about intimacy with a primary partner. He said, "Every relationship is a trial. The trick is to find the best trial that you can."[1] And at one level, I think that's true. To truly love another takes courage. Difficult moments will arise. So many of us were trained to assume that when someone became angry with us, we needed to be frightened for ourselves. That bad things would happen. Few of us understand that when someone is angry with us, it's because we matter to that person. We're *important* to that person. It's a myth that the opposite of love is hatred. That's not true; the opposite of love is indifference.

No good relationship is without its trials, and if we really love someone, and if we're in a relationship long enough, eventually conflicts will arise—and we need to be able to resolve these conflicts. We have to be willing to fight (fairly, of course), find resolution, and then move on. Sadly, however, it's at precisely this point that many people walk away from the relationship. They do not see that living through such conflicts is another way to put risk back into a relationship. It's scary to fight, of course, but once we resolve the conflict, we often feel closer than ever. Romance is based on feelings of intimacy, and where there's more intimacy, there's more romance. Conflict and courageous honesty are an invitation to greater intimacy.

Speaking the Truth

After a man I'll call "Keith" was divorced, he found that the new relationships he entered would only go so far—there was a level past which he couldn't seem to go. Eventually Keith sought professional help to look more deeply at some of the abuse issues that were part of his past. In so doing, he was able to redefine the pain that kept him from making a deeper commitment.

Keith is now happily married, but for more than six years, he was stuck in an on-and-off relationship with the woman who's now his wife. "I finally came to an impasse at which I realized that successful partnering is about two people who are really able to see that problems lie in themselves," explained Keith. "It made all the difference in the world to finally be able to finally let my wife see what I was struggling with." I can't count the number of divorced people I've spoken with in counseling who finally realize years after the breakup that the problem was not about their partners, it was about them—their unwillingness or inability to articulate their needs or concerns.

As individuals considering a relationship, we are faced with two decisions: The first is whether we can/want to enter into a relationship, and the second is with whom we want to have it. Successful relationships have far less to do with one's partner, and far more to do with one's level of self-awareness and willingness to commit; coming to this realization, though sometimes a lot of work, is possible. And once we get there, the rewards are wonderful.

The kind of courageous honesty Keith showed is not, however, something we're often taught. Quite the contrary, far too many of us were raised in families who lived by this famous phrase: "If you can't say something nice, don't say anything at all." Uttered by Thumper's mother to Bambi and Thumper in the famous 1942 Walt Disney movie *Bambi,* this phrase gave a whole generation of parents the idea that wonderfully paralleled the ideal families of *Donna Reed, Ozzie and Harriet,* and *Leave It to Beaver.* These television series depicted families in which everyone is always nice, no one is ever upset, nothing "messy" like divorce ever happens, and any problems that do crop up are basically comic rather than truly deep or tragic. Clearly *not* reality based!

Two points are important here. First, conflict between partners is inevitable. Even if we love someone deeply, sooner or later we're going to want to just throttle them! So somehow we have to get to a point where we can feel safe and comfortable enough to be truthful with one another. "If you can't say something nice, don't say anything at all" teaches people to be dishonest, because sometimes you simply must, if the relationship is to survive, say things to your partner about himself or herself, about yourself, and about the relationship that are painful and hard to hear.

When two people can speak at this level of truth, they know they're giving one another the unvarnished reality. By so doing we also let our partner know that we trust him or her—and the relationship—enough to speak the truth. Such actions build tremendous trust between partners because each knows that what they're dealing with is the truth. This deep level of honesty then becomes an ever-renewing well for risk taking and the intimacy that grows from it.

Here's the second point: The best way to be faithful to one's partner is to be faithful to oneself. By speaking truth, we become faithful to both ourselves and the other person. To understand more about this idea, we must jump back a few years to what I believe is the most important event in Twelve Step life since 1935 when Alcoholics Anonymous began: the creation of a program called "Recovering Couples Anonymous" (RCA).

Sacrilegious though it may sound, I believe that in many ways, Twelve Step programs have undermined relationships—though not intentionally—by failing to create a place where couples could come *together* to work the Twelve Steps. As we know from many, many family and marriage studies, when only one partner in a relationship seeks counseling about a family and marriage issue, the *relationship* problems often worsen. The same results often occur in Twelve Step recovery. Nearly ten years ago, couples started meeting together in RCA groups to remedy this common problem, and today countless couples credit these groups with providing the missing puzzle piece for their relationship's recovery.

How exactly has RCA made such a difference? Many couples immediately point to what happens when we talk together about a relationship problem. When the person to whom we're referring is sitting next to us, it's very difficult to put our own spin on the problem or to somehow put ourselves in a better light. There is no escaping reality, and, in such situations, a discipline of truth telling emerges.

RCA also encourages couples to view recovery as a three-legged stool: There's my recovery, your recovery, and *our* recovery *together*. This model is useful in viewing relationships too: There's my personal growth and challenges, your personal growth and challenges, and the challenges and growth of the relationship—three separate yet interdependent "beings," if you will.

As couples, we've been given a gift—the relationship—that we are to nurture together. Once we recognize that while each partner affects the health of the relationship, it has, in a sense, a life of its own too. From a Twelve Step perspective, RCA encourages partners to look at their relationship to discover the ways they have been powerless in their relationship over the stresses and systemic problems that reassert themselves over and over again. It's clear, too, that the couples who faired best in long-term studies of recovery are those who were surrounded by other couples who cared for them and with whom they could share problems and successes.[2] Couples have good relationships not because of chance, but because they have learned to build support for their coupleship.

Struggling relationships are usually characterized by a basic dysfunction that effectively blocks change and healing—what I call the "blame scenario." We all recognize it: One partner says, "These are all the things I've done for you, and still, after all this, look at how you treat me." The unspoken accusation is, "You're the bad person and I'm the good one."

RCA couples develop a weekly discipline that speaks directly to this scenario—one that any couple could benefit from following. It works like this. Each week, for example, I would make two lists. One list recounts the acts that I did which made life more difficult for my partner. The second list recounts the things my partner did that were gifts to me. Following this discipline encourages me to look specifically at *my* behavior in the relationship and its effect on my partner. Additionally, it forces me to focus on what I truly admire in my partner. Instead of blaming someone else for our problems, we focus instead on how we are living and affecting our partner.

I find that at times in my marriage, for example, I see things that I truly admire about my wife, but it's hard for me to actually tell her. Such moments, I suspect, happen in all relationships. We notice something we very much appreciate about our partner, but we never actually say, "This is remarkable." If we were courting that person, however, *of course* we'd say something. Again, this is where risk comes into play—the risk of putting ourselves on the line by opening up to another and showing who we are and what we're thinking. Sexuality truly thrives in such risk-taking environments.

The RCA weekly discipline reflects the spirit of Step Eight of the Twelve Steps in which we take an inventory of people whom we have harmed. In the RCA exercise, we begin to fearlessly take responsibility for the ways we've made life difficult for the people we love, particularly our partner. It's important to note, too, that in the Twelve Step program, all of the Steps are essentially part of one progressive inventory. With each Step, we add to what we've already accomplished, and in doing so move to a deeper level of growth and understanding. At Step Eight, we reach the final level of inventory by truly acknowledging to ourselves what we have done. We begin living with this in mind so as to create a new life. By reaching this level, we set the stage for living in a new environment in which we act authentically—and we find a new freedom to be sexual.

Love Addiction and Avoidance Addiction

In her groundbreaking book, *Facing Love Addiction*, author Pia Mellody describes what she has termed *love addiction* and *love avoidance*. Mellody outlines the dysfunctional patterns played out by Love Addicts and the unresponsive Avoidance Addicts to whom they are painfully and repeatedly drawn—patterns in which both partners deeply desire the kind of intimacy we are talking about while constantly fleeing from it. Relationships involving love addiction and love avoidance live, in a sense, at the opposite end of the spectrum. Examining them can help us understand and see more clearly the goal of healthy relationships and sexuality toward which we are moving.

A Love Addict, says Mellody, is someone who is dependent on, enmeshed with, and compulsively focused on taking care of another person. While this is often described as codependence, Mellody believes codependence is a much broader and more fundamental problem. Although being a codependent can lead some people into love addiction, not all codependents are Love Addicts. Mellody also states that although love addiction is found most often in female partners of sexual-romantic relationships, it's also possible for males to be Love Addicts.

Three characteristics sum up the major behavioral symptoms of a Love Addict.

1. Love Addicts assign a disproportionate amount of time, attention, and "value above themselves" to the person to whom they are addicted, and this focus often has an obsessive quality about it.
2. Love Addicts have unrealistic expectations for unconditional positive regard from the other person in the relationship.
3. Love Addicts neglect to care for or value themselves while they're in the relationship.

In addition to these three characteristics, Love Addicts are often in the grips of two principal fears. Their most conscious fear is abandonment. Love Addicts will tolerate almost anything to avoid being abandoned, the fear of which comes from such childhood experiences as abuse and neglect.

The irony is that while Love Addicts want to avoid abandonment and be connected to someone in a secure way, the close, demanding connection they try to establish is actually enmeshment rather than healthy intimacy, which they also fear, at least unconsciously. This denied fear also comes from the childhood experience of either physical or emotional abandonment, or both. Love Addicts did not experience enough intimacy from their abandoning caregivers to know how to be intimate in a healthy way.

Thus in adulthood, while Love Addicts often think they are intimate and are seeking an intimate relationship, they are, in fact, frightened by offers of healthy intimacy because they don't know what to do. When they reach a certain level of closeness, they often panic and do something to create distance between themselves and their partners again.

These two fears of abandonment and intimacy bring up the agonizing and self-defeating dilemma of the Love Addict. Love Addicts consciously want intimacy, but can't tolerate healthy closeness, so they must unconsciously choose a partner who cannot be intimate in a healthy way.

The painful patterns of love addiction are exhibited in relationships made up of two people, each of whom has certain distinct characteristics. One party is *focused on* the partner and the relationship; and the other, the Avoidance Addict, *tries to avoid* intimate connection within the relationship, usually through some type of addiction, such as to alcohol or other drugs.

Avoidance Addicts, the "model" partner for Love Addicts, have at least three characteristics that combine to result in avoiding intimacy.

1. Avoidance Addicts evade intensity within the relationship by creating intensity in activities (usually addictions) outside the relationship.
2. Avoidance Addicts avoid being known in the relationship in order to protect themselves from engulfment and control by the other person.
3. Avoidance Addicts avoid intimate contact with their partners by using a variety of processes called *distancing techniques*.

The Avoidance Addict's characteristics are most often seen in the male partner of romantic relationships between a man and a woman, although there are romantic relationships in which the reverse is true. It is also possible for one partner in a gay or lesbian relationship to have the characteristics of an Avoidance Addict. In addition, these characteristics can surface during other kinds of relationships—with children, parents or parents-in-law, a therapeutic client, or a close friend, to name just a few possibilities.

A fundamental trait of Avoidance Addicts' relationships is real abandonment. Avoidance Addicts don't share who they are in a realistic way with anyone. They conduct life from behind protective emotional walls, and like unseen puppeteers, they continually try to control the choices of other people with whom they are in partnership.

Avoidance Addicts consciously (and greatly) fear intimacy because they believe that they will be drained, engulfed, and controlled by it. In their families, family members had strong connections, but with too much intensity. This extremely intense connection is known as *enmeshment*.

In healthy families, the emotional connection between parent and child is like an emotional umbilical cord that goes from the parent to the child so that the parent, with a mature, stable sense of self, nurtures and supports the child.

Enmeshment is the opposite. The emotional connection between parent and child is also like an umbilical cord, except that the energy flows instead from the child to nurture the parent. A young teenage girl, for example, could be put into the role of confidant and friend to her mother. In this situation, the mother might share work problems, intimate details about her sex life, troubles with friends, and so on, and regularly tell the daughter that she is the mother's best and only true friend. Such enmeshed children are drained emotionally as they are used by their parent(s) for such nurturing acts as companionship, attention, and love.

In childhood, Avoidance Addicts were drained, engulfed, and controlled by somebody else's existence, and they don't want to go through that experience again. This childhood enmeshment experience created a deeply ingrained conviction that more intimacy will bring more misery, based on experience both with the original caregivers and with other Love Addict partners.

At the same time, Avoidance Addicts fear abandonment at some level. This fear is usually unconscious, although in some

Avoidance Addicts it is fairly close to the conscious level. The fear in adulthood stems from being abandoned as a child by the caregiver; when a child is forced to attend to the nurturance needs of the parent, the parent no longer meets the child's need for nurturing and care. Although abandonment is a less obvious experience for Avoidance Addicts than enmeshment, it is nevertheless real. Since Avoidance Addicts usually did not have contact in childhood with another human being who relieved the pain, fear, and emptiness of abandonment, they did not learn that a relationship can relieve the abandonment experiences. This unconscious fear of being abandoned nevertheless draws Avoidance Addicts *toward* relationships, even though they have great difficulty making a commitment to or connecting with a partner.

At an unconscious level, Avoidance Addicts recognize and are attracted to the Love Addict's strong fear of abandonment because Avoidance Addicts know that all they have to do to trigger their partner's fear of abandonment is threaten abandonment. Avoidance Addicts believe that being in control this way will allow them to escape being drained, engulfed, and controlled, and at a deeper level to avoid being abandoned themselves.

Avoidance Addicts thus have the same two fears as Love Addicts: intimacy and abandonment. The difference is that what is conscious for one is unconscious for the other. Love Addicts have a strong fear of abandonment and an unconscious fear of intimacy, which causes them unconsciously to pick someone who can't be intimate. Avoidance Addicts have a strong fear of intimacy, and yet also a deep underlying fear of abandonment. This keeps them on the front edge in relationships, where, for part of the time, they can feel powerful by meeting someone's needs without being engulfed.

I like to use the metaphor of a circle to describe relationships. Far too often, when one partner steps into the circle of the relationship, the other leaves. (The relationship of Love

Addict and Avoidance Addict is the quintessential example!) Then the one who left will step back into the circle, and the one already in the circle will leave. This process repeats itself until she (for example) becomes fed up and threatens to leave the relationship for good. Suddenly he is deeply in love, turns on the romance, and begs her to stay. She believes him enough to agree to stay and steps back into the circle—and then he "leaves" again.

In healthy relationships, both partners stay "in the circle." This is the goal we're striving toward, and it's with both partners in the circle of the relationship that we find ever-deepening intimacy and healthy sexuality.

Gay and Lesbian Partners

In chapters 10 and 12, Carl and Stephen talked from a gay perspective about sexual comfort and relationships. As Stephen says below, although there are far more similarities in the challenges gays/lesbians and straights experience in relationships, differences do exist.

> I believe now that family of origin has a far greater influence on problems in relationships than being gay or straight. I do think there are some gender-based differences between men and women. When two men come together in a relationship, the dynamics differ from a relationship of two women or from a male/female relationship.
>
> Carl and I, as well as other gays and lesbians we know, believe it's possible to identify gay, lesbian, and straight relationship norms—norms that are not identical. The sexuality of two men coming together is very different from that of a man and woman or two women coming together. Keep in mind that we're generalizing, of course, but when two men come together, the focus tends to be

more on sex than on relationship. For all our lesbian friends, the opposite seems to be the case: The bonding is based on the relationship, not the sex. With straight couples, these two forces seem to be more in balance—or perhaps we should say that there's more of a push–pull situation. Anonymous sex is fairly common in the gay culture, but not among lesbians. And it seems that gay relationships are shorter—we joke at our RCA group that we've been together for two years, but that's like ten for a straight couple.

There are differences in attitudes about monogamy too. It's not uncommon for gays to have encounters outside their primary partner relationship or to bring a third man into the relationship. In straight relationships, this just doesn't fit, especially for the women, it seems. The lesbian couples we know are very monogamous and family oriented. Of course, sex is a part of their relationships, but the relationship itself is far more important. We've seen very little interest among lesbian couples we know in bringing in another person. Gay men don't think monogamy has to be such a black-and-white issue.

Another difference exists over children and marriage. It seems that all the straight people we know are either married or thinking about getting married. Interest in marriage is changing now in the gay and lesbian community, and part of that change has to do, we think, with the possibility of being able to be legally married in some states. In addition, it seems like every lesbian couple we know has, or wants to have, children. Some gay couples want to have or do have kids, and perhaps the fact that marriage is becoming more possible accounts for this change.

When we decided to join RCA, we were very nervous. We knew we'd be the only gay couple in the group, and we came into it thinking that because we were gay, there wasn't much we could learn from the group and vice versa. Once we got past our heterophobia and realized we could share with the group in a loving, caring way, the similarities in our relationships and in our struggles became much more apparent. We discovered we could learn a lot from the other couples, and they from us. Of course, there are differences, but there are a lot more similarities.

Most of what goes on in a relationship is the same no matter who's involved—gays, lesbians, or straights. There are communication problems, the petty aggravations, the challenge of trying to blend two egos and two lives. Sexual preference does not affect this. It's very important for us to talk a lot about our relationship and the challenges we have, and RCA taught us to MAKE the time to do this in a structured way. People in recovery have a lot in common, and RCA helps us see this too. They are a great support to us.

We are both really trying to discover what healthy sexuality is for us—how to be sexual in a healthy way, and maybe this is what everybody's trying to do.

KEY QUESTIONS

Typically in workshops and in my counseling experience, the following question is asked when we talk about building relationships and living with a partner.

What is the difference between seduction and flirtation, and are either healthy?

Yes and no. My definition of seduction is high warmth with low intention. If a person touches you, for example, it could be a gesture of human friendship or it could be a sexual overture. The warmth of the gesture is clear; the intention behind it, however, is not. Seduction is inherently problematic because of the dishonesty involved.

Flirting is an exaggerated form of seduction in which the intent is very clear. The basic difference between seduction and flirtation is intent and the level of honesty involved. Flirting can be a playful and intimate part of both a courtship and a relationship. When a partner *says* "I'm going to seduce you," however, he or she has announced the intentions. There's no game playing behind it, and so it can truly be playful.

A. H. Maslow on Love in Self-Actualizing People

More than thirty years ago, psychologist Abraham H. Maslow undertook a study of a very specific group of people—those he termed healthy and self-actualizing.[3] These are individuals who live to their full human potential, achieving the full use of their talents and capabilities. Maslow studied all aspects of their lives, including their love relationships. His findings can act as a beacon to guide us as we strive to have healthier and more fulfilling love relationships.

One characteristic of love, says Maslow, is the absence of anxiety, and this is seen with exceptional clarity in healthy individuals. There is little question about the tendency to more and more complete spontaneity, to the dropping of defenses, to the dropping of roles, and of trying and striving in the relationship. As the self-actualized relationship continues, there is growing intimacy and honesty and self-expression. These people report that with a beloved person, it is possible to be oneself, to feel natural: "I can let my hair down." This honesty also includes allowing one's faults, weaknesses, and physical and psychological shortcomings to be freely seen by the partner.

There is much less tendency to put the "best foot forward" in the healthy love relationship, as well as much less maintenance of mystery and glamour, much less reserve and concealment and secrecy. This complete dropping of the guard definitely contradicts folk wisdom that says we have to be always at our best to maintain a relationship. Maslow further states that his data definitely contradict the age-old "intrinsic-hostility-between-the-sexes" theory. This notion of intergender hostility and suspicion, the tendency to identify with one's own gender in alliance against the other, even the very phrasing itself of "opposite sex," is definitely not found in self-actualizing people.

Self-actualizing love is based on a healthy acceptance of the self and of others. There tends to be a rather easy relationship with the opposite sex, along with casual acceptance of the phenomenon of being attracted to other people; at the same time, these individuals do rather less about this attraction than other people. In addition, their talk about sex is considerably more free and casual and unconventional than the average person's. This seems to indicate an acceptance of the facts of life which, together with the more intense and profound and satisfying love relationship, makes it less *necessary* [Maslow's emphasis] to seek for compensatory or neurotic sex affairs outside the marriage.

According to Maslow, another characteristic of love in healthy people is that they make no sharp differentiation between the roles and personalities of the genders. That is, they do not assume the female is passive and the male aggressive, whether in sex, love, or anything else. These people are so certain of their maleness or femaleness that they do not mind taking on some of the cultural aspects of the opposite-gender roles.

It is especially noteworthy, says Maslow, that they can be both active and passive lovers, which was clearest in physical lovemaking. In self-actualizing people, the gender "dichotomies" are resolved, and the individual becomes both active and passive, both selfish and unselfish, both masculine and feminine, both self-interested and self-effacing.

Erich Fromm in his book *Man for Himself* writes, "Genuine love is an expression of productiveness and implies care, respect, responsibility and knowledge. It is not an 'affect' in the sense of being affected by somebody, but an active striving for the growth and happiness of the loved person, rooted in one's own capacity to love."[4]

All serious writers on the subject of ideal or healthy love have stressed the affirmation of the other's individuality, the eagerness for the growth of the other, the essential respect for his or her individuality and unique personality. This is confirmed very strongly by Maslow's observation of self-actualizing people, who have in unusual measure the rare ability to be pleased rather than threatened by a partner's triumphs. A most impressive example of this respect is the ungrudging pride of such people in their spouse's achievements, even when outshining their own. Another is the absence of jealousy.

Self-actualizing people acknowledge and respect others as separate and autonomous individuals. They will not casually use another or control another or disregard another's wishes.

ISSUES

Many sexual anorexics struggle with the following issues in reference to partnership. Some of these issues have been explored at greater length in this or previous chapters; for those which have not, a brief discussion is included here. Read the issues carefully, noting the ones that apply to you. Then use those issues as discussion points with your partner and/or fair witnesses.

❈ Difficulty making appropriate partner choices.

Whom do we pick to be in a relationship with us? Who's "right" for us? Making this decision causes much trouble for some people, and they simply have difficulty making appropriate partner choices. We've all seen partners that we and their other friends knew were simply not a good match. The relationship likely started out well, degenerated over some time, and eventually ended badly—and we all saw it coming from the start.

Making good decisions about whom to start a relationship with requires, first of all, some level of self-awareness and self-knowledge. What are your "assets and liabilities"; in other words, what do you have to offer someone, and what areas are you still working on? Pay attention to the kind of partner to whom you're attracted. Is that kind of person good for you? Some women with backgrounds of childhood abuse, for example, regularly find themselves attracted to abusive men. Conversely, look at the kind of people you seem to attract. Can you discover any patterns?

And who *is* right for us? Abraham Maslow's research on love in healthy people[5] gives us some insight into the answer. (See the sidebar "A. H. Maslow on Love in Self-Actualizing People" for more on this topic.) As the people in his study grew more mature, they were less attracted by such characteristics as *handsome, good dancer, breasts, tall,* and *handsome,* and spoke more of *compatibility, goodness, decency, good companionship,* and *considerateness.*

Two common theories about partner attractions were contradicted by Maslow's data. One is that opposites attract, and the other that like marries like. In healthy people, like *does* attract like with respect to character traits such as honesty, sincerity, kindliness, and courage. The more external and superficial characteristics—such as income, class, education, religion, appearance, and nationality—are far less relevant. Self-actualizing people are not threatened by strangeness, but rather intrigued by it.

As for opposites attracting, Maslow found this true to the extent that he saw one partner honestly admiring skills and talents that he or she did not possess. Such abilities make a potential partner *more* rather than less attractive for those with a positive, strong sense of self.

Maslow further found that the dichotomy of "head versus heart" is nonexistent too. The people with whom his subjects fell in love were selected by *either* head or heart. That is, they were *intuitively, sexually,* and *impulsively* attracted to people who were right for them by cold, intellectual, clinical calculation. Their appetites agreed with their judgments and were synergistic rather then antagonistic.

✿ Being blocked in initiating a relationship.
Many people know what kind of person they want, but have extreme difficulty initiating a relationship. Time and again, they pass up chances to enter relationships with good people because of this fear.

✿ Being vulnerable to victim/victimization scenarios of the past.
Abuse victims can be very vulnerable to falling into abusive relationships. The victim/victimizing scenario of the past can start off as a romantic relationship and end up as a war. Additionally, if individuals have been in abusive relationships, fear of abuse recurring can paralyze them. What's more, they find it difficult to imagine that something better can happen.

✿ Facing problems in sustaining and renewing an existing partnership.
I have often sat in my office and listened to couples talk about their relationship problems, only to finally turn to them and say, "You know, there really is nothing in this relationship that's not fixable—if you really want to do it." The difficulty they encounter is their inability to be honest enough with one another to renew and sustain their partnership.

❋ Dealing with sexual betrayal, either as victim or betrayer. Whether we've been the betrayed or the betrayer, our relationship will suffer. Rebuilding and sustaining trust and honesty with our partner will be difficult.

❋ Repeating the same sexual scenarios over and over again. Sadly, some people, because of being victimized in the past, find themselves in the same abusive sexual scenario over and over again. They compulsively repeat their bad relationships until, with help, they recognize that they do indeed deserve more.

❋ Exploring how the principles of healthy sexuality can change rules of abandonment.
This issue speaks to the core of this chapter. In my younger years, I found that when meeting and dating women, I would think, "How can I impress this woman so she'll be interested in me and like me?" The more appropriate question to ask, of course, would have been, "What is it like to be me in this woman's presence?"

In other words, I need only to focus on being exactly who I am—nothing more and nothing less—because when I do this, a very different set of dynamics engages. If I am fully myself and this woman is interested in me, then she's interested in the *real* me, and immediately I can trust in this relationship. I don't have to live in fear of abandonment.

When people hold up a false ego for others to see, with the real person hidden, the distance between the two will always be one's anxiety. We can't help but worry that this person will discover who we really are behind the false self we're projecting. Be yourself, and look for a person with whom you can fully be yourself.

❋ Dealing with sexual exploitation.
Sexual exploitation, whether perpetrated by parents, caregiver,

or professional person, creates a serious breach of trust, one with far-reaching consequences. It is very important to understand the effect of this experience. Likewise, it's important to understand that not all people will take advantage of us in this manner, and to learn how to have a trusting relationship.

🌺 Overcoming sexualized conflicts.
Some couples have organized their whole relationship around sexualized conflict. They get into an argument and then they get into bed, for example. Or they have a fight in bed, they get out and have a bigger fight, and then they get back into bed. The partners rebound between fighting and sex. Needless to say, this very destructive and powerful cycle must be broken before a healthy relationship can be created.

It *IS* Possible to Learn How to Love Better!

It's not at all unusual for therapists working with couples to hear one or both partners complain about not feeling loved by the other, or at least not loved enough. In particular, these feelings interfere with couples' attempts to improve their sexual relationship.

"I just can't do sex unless I feel loved!" "Without love, sex is so mechanical!" "Please help us to do it with love!" Such lamentations bemoaning sex without love echo on. But is it possible to learn to love better? To break love into specific behaviors that couples could actually practice that would help them feel more loved? The work of J. Richard Conkerly and Kathleen McClaren shows that the answer is an unequivocal yes![6]

Over the years, numerous studies and much anecdotal evidence have shown that people can, in fact, learn to love better.[7] In addition, learning how to better show one's love can dramatically affect the success couples have in improving and remaining satisfied with their sexual relationships.

Here are eight love behaviors we can learn.

1. *Affirming love behaviors:* acts that show emotional and moral support for the person we love; that show we enjoy and appreciate the idiosyncratic side of our partner; that show respect for and have a high value of the person we love.

2. *Expressing love behaviors:* tones of voice, gestures, postures, and facial expressions that show our love.

3. *Verbal love behaviors:* words, pet names, and phrases that show expressions of love.

4. *Self-disclosing love behaviors:* acts and words revealing intimate facts and unique aspects; being open and vulnerable.

5. *Tolerating love behaviors:* acts showing an acceptance of the less-pleasant aspects of the other—and doing so without judging the partner.

6. *Tactile love behaviors:* physical contact demonstrating loving affection and loving sexuality.

7. *Object/gift love behaviors:* giving gifts that demonstrate how much we care for our partner.

8. *Receptional love behaviors:* acts and words that show that we appreciate it when any of the previous behaviors were done for us.

Interestingly, however, early studies showed that focusing only on teaching the above eight categories of behaviors resulted in little success among couples. The ultimate key to success involved adding what researchers called "reception skills." These include the following:

1. Actively identifying and focusing on each expression of love as it is shown by your partner;

2. Avoiding discounting (putting down or ignoring) the expression of love when you notice it; and

3. Giving appropriate comments that show you did notice and appreciated the expression of love.

Partners

In other words, it's not enough to just express these love behaviors. *If you receive love, you have to let your partner know clearly that you noticed and appreciated it!* Don't assume your partner knows you appreciate what he or she has done; TELL your partner that you do! Be specific too.

This is simply invaluable, striking, and wonderfully hopeful information. Rather than thinking we have to remain stuck in old sexual patterns and live the same kind of sexual scenarios over and over again, we can choose to do something else.

Here's a way of looking at love and its composite elements that's admittedly not too romantic, but if these behaviors are learned and practiced in your relationship, romance is just about guaranteed to return. This gives new meaning to the expression "making love."

TASKS

Once you've read the sidebar "It *IS* Possible to Learn How to Love Better!" then complete the following exercise.

Building an Enduring Relationship

Listed here are the eight behaviors of love and three "reception behaviors" that can help partners build an enduring relationship. Below each is a scale on which you and your partner can rate yourselves. (1 = needs to learn and do more; 10 = nothing more need be done.) When you're finished, use the results to see what areas each of you would like to improve.

Write a plan on how you'll proceed—and have fun with this. Talk at least weekly about how you're both doing—and how it feels to give and receive these "love behaviors."

1. Affirming love behaviors: acts that show emotional and moral support for the person you love; that show you enjoy and appreciate the idiosyncratic side of your partner; that show respect for and have a high value of the person you love.

   I   2   3   4   5   6   7   8   9   10

2. Expressing love behaviors: tones of voice, gestures, postures, and facial expressions that show your love.

   I   2   3   4   5   6   7   8   9   10

3. Verbal love behaviors: words, pet names, and phrases that show expressions of love.

   I   2   3   4   5   6   7   8   9   10

4. Self-disclosing love behaviors: acts and words revealing intimate facts and unique aspects; being open and vulnerable.

   I   2   3   4   5   6   7   8   9   10

5. Tolerating love behaviors: acts showing an acceptance of the less-pleasant aspects of your partner—and doing so without judging the partner.

   I   2   3   4   5   6   7   8   9   10

6. Tactile love behaviors: physical contact demonstrating loving affection and loving sexuality.

   I   2   3   4   5   6   7   8   9   10

7. Object/gift love behaviors: giving gifts that demonstrate how much you care for your partner.

   I   2   3   4   5   6   7   8   9   10

8. Receptional love behaviors: acts and words that show that you appreciate it when your partner did any of the previous behaviors for you.

I   2   3   4   5   6   7   8   9   10

RECEPTION SKILLS:

1. Actively identifying and focusing on each expression of love as it is shown by your partner.

I   2   3   4   5   6   7   8   9   10

2. Avoiding discounting (putting down or ignoring) the expression of love when you notice it.

I   2   3   4   5   6   7   8   9   10

3. Giving appropriate comments that show you did notice and appreciated the expression of love.

I   2   3   4   5   6   7   8   9   10

PLANNING

This chapter introduced you to the RCA writing discipline. Each week for the next month or so, follow this discipline. Each week, you and your partner should make two lists.

One list should recount the acts you did that made life more difficult for your partner. In doing this list, focus only on your behavior in the relationship and its effect on your partner. The second list should recount the things your partner did that were gifts to you.

Once the two of you have completed your lists, share them with one another.

IN YOUR JOURNAL

Start each morning by writing your "daily pages." In addition, since this chapter focuses on partners, focus on your partnership, keeping in mind what we have talked about.

Intimacy Dimensions

Here's another way to look at your ability to be intimate. On the chart that follows, you will find in the left column qualities of healthy intimacy, while in the right column are qualities of unhealthy intimacy. You will also find that the concept of intimacy has been divided into seven dimensions, or categories.

In the *Initiative* category, for example, a person who has the ability to be intimate in a healthy way will be able to reach out to others, risk expressions of caring (to say, "I love you" or "I missed you"), invite others to share activities, share and talk about their problems with others, and express their desires and needs to another. Those who have problems with intimacy are passive and isolated, unable to ask for what they need, assume the role of victim (they feel they have little or no power), and often feel as though no one cares for them.

Look over this chart with your partner. When you're finished, you may want to work on some of the dimensions of intimacy that are a problem for you. If you do, it's important to be very clear about which ones you're going to work on, and about how you will address each issue. For example, perhaps you and your partner decided that in the intimacy category entitled "Play," you want to dance more. First, ask yourselves what specific steps you will need to take to make dance a greater part of your life. You might check in the phone book for places that teach dancing, for example. You could look in the newspaper for clubs that have music you like and could dance to. Remember that your reticence to dance may stem from embarrassing childhood experiences about dancing, or it may relate to a core belief that you won't be able to dance well enough for your partner, and that your partner will leave you because of this. Share your feelings with your partner as you become aware of them. This is another way to be courageous in your relationship and to take healthy risks.

INTIMACY DIMENSIONS
Initiative

Healthy intimacy

I will call on others
I reach out to others
I risk expressions of caring
I invite others to share activities
I share problems/concerns
I'm able to express desire and
  attraction

Unhealthy intimacy

I'm passive
I'm isolated
I act like a victim
Things just happen to me
I have no control over my life
I always feel abandoned

Presence

Healthy intimacy

I initiate activities
I meet others, I listen
I pay attention to others and the
  world around me
I have explicit reactions to people
  and events
I'm open with my feelings
I take part in activities with
  others regularly
I notice details

Unhealthy intimacy

My feelings are constricted
I'm unavailable to others because
  of feelings of shame
I deflect both positive and negative
  attention away from me, believing I don't deserve either
My obsessions block attention that
  might come my way

Closure

Healthy intimacy

I finalize arrangements
I acknowledge and care about
  others
I acknowledge others who desire
  my time or who are attracted
  to me
I work to conclude things
I express thanks

Unhealthy intimacy

I make everything into a crisis
I'm out of control; so overextended
  that loose ends are everywhere
  in my life
I avoid closure, I can't resolve problems or concerns

Vulnerability

Healthy intimacy

I share problems
I share my process of thinking
and feelings.
I involve others in decisions
I reveal myself and share who I
am with others
I talk about myself

Unhealthy intimacy

I keep my thoughts private
My decision-making process is
private
My internal dialogues are secret
and unshared, but I still rely on
them.

Nurturance

Healthy intimacy

I make caring statements, and I
care for others
I'm empathetic
I support others
I feel life
I make suggestions
I help others in need
I provide feedback to others
I let other people know that they
have value

Unhealthy intimacy

I always try to take care of others
I don't allow others to have
feelings
I discount or diminish others
and/or their effort

Honesty

Healthy intimacy

I acknowledge my positive and
negative feelings
I'm clear about my priorities and
values
I'm specific about disagreements

Unhealthy intimacy

I don't acknowledge that I have
deep feelings
I seldom, if ever, express my preferences
I disguise anger in order to have
sex
I rely on third parties to communicate with my partner

Play

Healthy intimacy

I can see humor in life
I put effort into leisure time
I celebrate joyful events
I'm willing to dance
I explore new ventures with
others
I like to smell flowers
I enjoy children
I laugh easily

Unhealthy intimacy

I'm compulsively busy
I miss significant events
I have a grim demeanor—a "life's-a-
mess" attitude
I don't experiment in life
I'm compulsive about hobbies

A CLOSING EXERCISE

The closing exercise asks you and your partner to evaluate yourselves and one another. Remember, this exercise offers a wonderful opportunity for you to discover your strengths and weaknesses, as well as a chance for you and your partner to compare your perceptions of yourselves and one another.

In addition to filling out the rating scales, it will be helpful to do the following:

- Once you have filled out your scales, share the results with your fair witnesses.
- After your partner has finished, talk about your partner's perceptions too. They may differ from yours and/or those of your fair witnesses.
- If significant discrepancies exist, note them and then return to your fair witnesses to look into them more carefully.

As you work on these scales, try not to become defensive if the perceptions your partner or your fair witnesses have of you differ from your own perceptions of yourself. Let these differences—and the reasons for them—be a source of information for all of you.

If you are not currently in a relationship, ask one of your fair witnesses (therapist, sponsor, anorexia group member, Twelve Step support group member, or RCA group member, for example) to work through the scales with you.

Part 1: Focus on You

Is your "guard down" with your partner? Do you tell your partner what you appreciate about him or her? What angers you? What do you want from the relationship? Do you practice "love behaviors"? How much work do you need to do on your partnership?

Using a circle, rate yourself on the scale below. (1 = low skills, need much work; 10 = high skills, need no further work.)

Next, ask your partner to rate your partnership skills and abilities. Have your partner use a square to rate you.

I   2   3   4   5   6   7   8   9   10

Part 2: Focus on Your Partner

On this second scale, ask your partner to rate his or her skills and ability in this area. Is your partner's "guard down" with you? Does your partner tell you what he or she appreciates about you? What angers your partner? What does your partner want from the relationship? Does your partner practice "love behaviors"? How much work does your partner need to do on your partnership?

Have your partner use a circle to rate himself or herself.

Next, you rate your partner's partnerships skills and ability. Use a square to do so.

I   2   3   4   5   6   7   8   9   10

Nurturing—
We learn to trust and to open our lives to experience.

Sensuality—
Through our senses, we interact with the world around us
and become connected to it.

Self-Image—
We learn that we are good and lovable.

Self-Definition—
We develop a relationship with ourselves and come to trust
ourselves. We are trustworthy.

Comfort—
We learn that we can trust others.

Knowledge—
With the acceptance of ourselves and others, we seek to grow
as people.

Relationships—
Based on what we have learned, we make the leap of trying to
live in new ways.

Partners—
We take responsibility for ourselves.

14

NONGENITAL SEX

WHEN WE MENTION SEX, the first thing that comes to most of our minds is "the Big O"—orgasm. How men can delay theirs; how women can achieve theirs. How good it was, and on and on. With all the focus on the culmination of intercourse, it's easy to assume that orgasm is the most important part of sex. Is it?

When people are actually asked what the best part of sex is, in overwhelming numbers they say it's such activities as kissing, holding, fondling—in other words, nongenital sex. And yes, *both* men and women say this.

Despite such strong attitudes about nongenital sex, studies also show that as many as fortyfive percent of couples take less than ten minutes to prepare for intercourse. Many of us skip over the best part of sex! Nongenital sex is by all accounts the most highly regarded and appreciated dimension of sexuality, yet one of the most neglected. Orgasm, I like to say, is a lot like Christmas. It's a fun and intense holiday that goes by very quickly, but it's all the time and preparation that make Christmas the experience it is!

I'm always a little dismayed to see how quickly new relationships progress to genital sex; if we skip over nongenital sex during courtship, we may have difficulty reclaiming it once we are in a long-term relationship. For similar reasons, I have even-greater concerns about young teens becoming sexual.

When these youngsters move quickly to intercourse, they lose the opportunity to acclimatize to their sexual feelings—and they begin a pattern of hurried sex (to avoid detection by parents or other adults) that can carry into their adult lives.

People who have visited Disneyland and Disney World may be familiar with the E-tickets these parks offer. (I know you're wondering why we've gone from orgasm to entertainment parks, but bear with me!) E-tickets allow their purchasers immediate access to all rides in the park. There's no standing in line, no preparation—you can just walk to the head of the line, get on the ride, and go until you drop. Immediate gratification, of course—but at a rather high price. E-tickets run about $600.

When it comes to sex, too many people have what I like to call "E-ticket" personalities, particularly addicts, codependents, and survivors of abuse. E-ticket folks are constantly searching for stimulation—and the more immediate the better. They are not particularly interested in process and preparation, and this approach holds true for them in sex too. They head straight for the Big O, to heck with the rest. But the price they pay is high—they miss out on the best part of sex.

Celibacy Contract

In working with people who are compulsively nonsexual as well as with those who are compulsively sexual, sex therapists and others in the addictions field have discovered an intervention that can help not only these people but also any couple struggling with a sexual relationship—a period of abstinence from sex.

I know that on the surface, a period of celibacy may seem a rather odd therapy. When it's "prescribed" for couples who are struggling with sex, many immediately ask, "How can not doing it at all help with our problem?" When, however, the possibility of genital sex is off-limits for a time, couples are forced to explore being with each other as companions. They have to rely on other means to express feelings and affection. Often they quickly discover that the mate who was boring, uninteresting, unattractive, and unsexy suddenly becomes flirtatious, interesting, and sexually enticing.

An abstinence contract can also help people who have more deep-seated and difficult problems, such as sexual anorexics, sex addicts, and their partners. As sex addicts' lives become further out of control sexually, for example, their partners will often close off and become compulsively nonsexual. A partner will tell the therapist that she hasn't had a sexual thought in years, but when she learns that her guy is working on a celibacy contract, suddenly he becomes overwhelmingly attractive to her. He's not safe walking down the treatment center halls!

So then we have to ask ourselves, if this woman hasn't had a sexual thought in years, where did all these feelings of sexuality come from? She had them all the time, of course, but the situation in which she was living led her to suppress them. Therapists have found that for both the sex addict and the sexual anorexic, guaranteeing a time away from sex is very, very effective. It can remove the *pressure* to be sexual, thereby allowing the partners to step back, become reacquainted with each other, and work through their difficulties.

JUNE AND BILL'S STORY

The story of a couple I'll call "June and Bill," who are in their third and second marriages, respectively, illustrates the value of a sexual time-out. June, whose father was alcoholic, lived in an extremely wealthy and extremely dysfunctional family. One of the messages June repeatedly received while growing up was that she was worthwhile only when she was sexy and provoking. For this behavior, June was rewarded by her father with much approval and support (a covert form of incest, I might add)—and by her mother with humiliation and rejection. During her teen years, June became progressively more promiscuous and later worked as a high-class prostitute.

June eventually recognized that she had a big problem and entered therapy. She had by this time also met Bill, who was chemically dependent and a sex addict. While June and Bill were courting, sex was hot, passionate, and immediate. After their marriage, however, Bill's sex addiction and acting out brought the relationship to a breaking point. Both Bill and June realized that they needed help to solve their problems.

One pattern had emerged in their relationship: June found that she would shut down emotionally and sexually whenever Bill approached her sexually—even when showing just the slightest hint of attraction to her. This was the same man June was constantly trying to seduce while they were courting! What had happened is this: June began to realize that in order to maintain her relationship with Bill, she had to be sexual with him. This, however, triggered all those old feelings about her father and her need to be sexy to maintain his approval. As a result, not long into her marriage with Bill, June switched from sexual-addiction behaviors (promiscuity) to sexual anorexia. June now hated *anything* to do with sexuality. Eventually, June's therapist urged her and Bill to agree to a celibacy contract.

June and Bill found that a period of sexual abstinence allowed them to open themselves to their feelings. In the past, they had used sex or the avoidance of sex as a way to medicate feelings of depression, loneliness, and pain. Once sex was out of the picture, those suppressed feelings could resurface along with the underlying problems. Without any expectations to perform sexually, Bill and June were free to explore solutions to their problems.

The Role of Nongenital Sex

Thus far in this book, we have discussed the importance of nurturing and sensuality, of a positive sense of self, of knowing who we are as men and women, of self-definition, of increasing our knowledge of our bodies. Each constitutes a major dimension of our sexuality—and *none* of them involve genital touch.

During a vacation from sex, couples can, without pressure, explore these dimensions in themselves. Often they first discover a renewed interest in one another. A deeper level of exploration occurs, creating greater intimacy. With intimacy, trust emerges along with playfulness. Gone is the sexual anorexic's ever-present fear that the partner will want to be sexual. The partners instead focus on the myriad ways they can connect with themselves and one another. They can at last relax and just enjoy one another.

At the same time, the partners can work on their sexuality. From a therapist, they can receive step-by-step assignments that include focusing on touch, massage, mutual sensory exploration, and more. (See the exercises in this chapter.) They begin to reacquaint themselves with their sexuality—awakening long-forgotten feelings and sensations. As is so often the case, June, too, discovered that sexuality does not have as much to do with a partner as it does with our relationship to our *own* selves and sexuality.

We have abandoned part of ourselves by focusing only on genital sex, and now we have the opportunity to remedy this situation. We are taking the actions needed to repair our relationships, actions that are in the spirit of the Ninth Step. We are in a sense making amends to our partner and to ourselves for what we've done. We are working to make both ourselves and our relationship whole.

It's not unusual for couples to find a time of celibacy so useful that they voluntarily agree to repeat it three or four years later. Again, they say, they are reminded of the value of nongenital contact—the importance of focusing on sensuality rather than orgasm. The second time around, the experience often has a new quality about it—because the partners have matured and become wiser. Lessons learned differ from those in the first experience, but are no less valuable. They find their relationship once again revitalized.

The Importance of Touch

Simple physical touch is the most basic way we have to show each other warmth and affection. Any kind of loving touch, from hugging a friend to cradling a baby to caressing one's romantic partner, conveys a powerful message of caring to the person who receives it.

The need to touch and be touched is inside all of us, beginning from the time we are born. Indeed, studies show that babies who are lovingly handled fare much better than those who receive little or no physical contact. Our need for contact continues throughout our lives.

Why do so many people place little emphasis on touch when it is such an important human need? A lot depends on our upbringing and the ways of our culture. North Americans, unlike many Latin cultures, for example, are not encouraged to engage in frequent nonsexual touching. Men in particular have difficulty in accepting touch. As children, boys tend to receive much less touching than girls because some parents mistakenly believe that affectionate physical contact with a son will diminish his masculinity. Many men thus grow up feeling uneasy about touch, particularly receiving it.

Some men who feel uncomfortable about this kind of physical contact only touch when they want to make love with their partners. When this happens, the woman may feel her partner doesn't really love her, but only desires her for sex. And both partners miss out on the full range of satisfactions that occur with a variety of touch: the affectionate warmth of an embrace, a reassuring hand on the shoulder, the sensual (rather than sexual) stroking of a back rub or massage. Men who equate touching with sex may focus all their attention on their partners' sexual parts, but many women crave overall body contact, with plenty of stroking and caressing, in order to become aroused. This doesn't mean the man is to blame, but that his partner needs to tell him what she wants.

Authors Mary Ann Klausner and Bobbie Hasselbring in their

book *Aching for Love* looked carefully at children who grew up in alcoholic or otherwise dysfunctional families. They discovered that many of these children are touch deprived. Children living without the important emotional intimacy and physical nurturing that children in healthy families receive greatly crave human touch. As they grow older, one of the mistakes they often make is concluding that the only way to meet this need is through sex. When they are sexual, however, they often come away disappointed because it wasn't sex they really wanted.

When partners, for whatever the reason, are unable or unwilling to touch one another, it usually indicates an underlying problem between them. Once they recognize this situation, they may choose to seek help through a marriage or sex therapist.

As part of therapy, sex therapists often employ what are called "sensate-focus exercises." *Sensate* refers to the senses; thus, sensate-focus is to concentrate attention on the senses. These exercises teach couples to give and receive pleasure through touch—but without a sense of pressure or demand to engage in sex. Pioneered by Masters and Johnson in the 1970s, they are designed to disrupt the patterns of performance anxiety that often inhibit a couple's sexual enjoyment. (Examples of such exercises appear later in this chapter.)

Masters and Johnson point out that for many men and women, "sensate-focus sessions represent the first opportunity they have ever had to 'think and feel' sensuously and at leisure, without intrusion upon the experience by any demand." Without worrying about ejaculation and orgasm, couples are liberated to explore one another sensually.

Today, with so many published guides on how to make love, "sensate-focus may seem a bit tame," say the writers of *Sex over Forty*. "But many couples have simply forgotten how important it is to touch each other, to express warmth and tenderness through their fingers. The entire body is like an instrument available for tuning: the ears, the neck, the small of the back, the fingertips, even the toes. Once a couple's capacity to give pleasure through touch is rekindled, they will be more receptive to fondling of the penis and clitoris and to the consummation of their passion in sexual intercourse."[1]

KEY QUESTIONS

Typically in workshops and in my counseling experience, the following questions are asked when we talk about nongenital sex.

If sex is not exciting or dangerous, it does not work for me. What do I do?
This question speaks to appropriate risk taking. The risks of anonymous sex or affairs, for example, may create excitement and danger, but they are ultimately unfulfilling and eventually lead to self-destruction. We need to redefine the risks we take. As mentioned in our discussions about relationships, what sustains romance is an ongoing sense of risk—the risk that comes with being completely honest with ourselves and with our partner. This leads to the following question.

I don't even know how to talk about what I really want because it will seem weird to my partner if I do.
Again, at issue is our ability to take the risk needed to be honest with our partner about what would feel good for us. What would we like? How would we like to be touched? What would our partner really enjoy? Again, the risk and excitement come in putting ourselves on the line and expressing what we want. (Refer to the exercises and resources on sexual communication in chapter 10.)

ISSUES

Many sexual anorexics struggle with the following issues in reference to nongenital sex. Some of these issues have been explored at greater length in this or previous chapters; for those which have not, a brief discussion is included here. Read the issues carefully, noting the ones that apply to you. Then use those issues as discussion points with your partner and/or fair witnesses.

❦ Touching as a trigger for abuse memories.
For those who have been abused, touch can, even in the context of a loving, supportive relationship, trigger past painful memories. Certain parts of the body or certain ways of being approached remind abuse survivors of inappropriate ways they were touched. In such cases, touch becomes a cue to shut down. They may not be able to move much beyond the preliminary stages in their arousal cycle—or even experience desire—before touch causes them to shut down.

People with backgrounds of adult or childhood deprivation and/or abuse need to learn how to touch without worrying about where it will lead (see the sensate-focus exercises). They also need to practice trying to stay right in the moment, which can create an opportunity to learn to enjoy touch, and to understand what touch actually means for them.

❦ Using touch as a way to acclimatize oneself to more fearful levels of sexual contact.

❦ Experiencing difficulty in expressing needs.
As discussed in chapter 6, if we have difficulty nurturing ourselves, we'll likewise have difficulty expressing our needs. It is fine to have these needs met, but we'll seldom see that happen if we simply wait for others to guess what they are.

To say what we would really like our partner to do for us requires taking a risk. Maybe when we made such requests in our past, we were ignored or shamed. Perhaps as children our needs were ignored. But that doesn't mean this will still happen today.

Or perhaps we just don't really know how to ask for what we need and like because we've simply never done so before. Again, we have to take the risk, or nothing will ever change. It's very important for both our sexual relationship and our overall relationship to talk about our needs.

❋ Being compulsive about being noncompulsive.

Once we discover how compulsive we tend to be, some of us try to remedy the situation by being compulsively noncompulsive. We fall into a pattern in which we always try to do things differently. Or we become compulsive about trying to be spontaneous, never making any plans, and so on. So often addicts live in the extremes; addicts need to strive to find and live in the middle ground. Balance is the key here.

❋ Practicing sexual perfectionism.

Efforts at sexual perfection stem from an attitude that there's a "right" way to do sex. What's actually right grows out of taking the risk to be honest about what you and your partner like and feel comfortable doing. And that can change from day to day, depending on our moods and feelings and bodies. It's important to let go of performance standards. No one is grading you here! If you and your partner are happy with what's happening, it's fine. If you're not, talk about how you can make it better. Remember, too, that some of the most amazingly fun times happen when you make "mistakes." This is where it's really fine to just be yourself; don't try to fit some pattern or image of what you think sex should be.

As mentioned, the highest-rated sexual activity is nongenital touch, yet 45 percent of couples spend less than ten minutes preparing for intercourse. Sexual anorexics are particularly vulnerable to skipping the best part because of their anxiety about performance. Our goal is to reduce this anxiety by focusing on nongenital expression. Anorexics must also gather the courage to be imperfect in their sexual expression.

✱ Experiencing the sexual double bind.
Some people place themselves in a sexual double bind that says the only good sex is "stolen" or "illicit" and therefore must be hurried. If it is good, it has to be bad, and therefore rushed.

✱ Focusing on sexual management by objectives (MBOs).
MBOs suggests that end goals are more important than the process. Don't focus on objectives; when we do, we miss the process. Remember our Christmas metaphor!

TASKS

Human beings touch one another in a wide variety of ways, most of which are not sexual at all. To see how different touch experiences interrelate, imagine a continuum of sensual touch ranging from less to more sexual kinds of touch. In her ground-breaking book *The Sexual Healing Journey*, sex therapist Wendy Maltz describes such a continuum, from holding, rocking together, and playful touch; through hugging, kissing, and soothing stroking; to massage and sexual pleasuring. As Maltz points out, we ideally experience and learn to enjoy touch as infants, children, adolescents, and adults in stages that essentially follow this continuum. Sexual abuse and severe neglect interrupt or abort this process by deleting critical stages of touch experiences or rearranging the order of the stages. The result is that the abuse victim is denied the opportunity to develop a foundation of pleasurable touch experiences upon which to emotionally and psychologically organize and interpret his or her touch experiences as an adult.

The good news is, however, that abuse survivors can still build that foundation of touch experiences, even as adults, by performing certain exercises that help them to "relearn" touch. This "relearning" is done by recreating the continuum described above with therapeutically designed touch exercises. (While you may choose to vary slightly the specific stages of the continuum to fit your needs or those of your partner, make sure it allows for a progression from nonsexual to more sexual kinds of touch.) Chapter 10 of *The Sexual Healing Journey* provides detailed instructions for several exercises for relearning touch, from drawing pictures on your partner's back with your finger, to having your partner shampoo your hair, and on up the continuum to partner massage. I highly recommend that you obtain a copy of *The Sexual Healing Journey* and practice the exercises described in chapter 10 of that book, beginning with the "sensory basket" exercise (p. 263) and continuing through the "reclaiming your body" exercise (p. 276). You may also do the "body massage, with partner" exercise described on pp. 280-281.[2]

PLANNING

When we relearn touch, we increase our ability to experience pleasure on our own and with a trusted partner.

As you do the exercises for relearning touch, you begin to acquire a new, healthier collection of memories about touch. In the future, repeating these exercises may help solve specific problems with sexual functioning—or just reinforce what you've learned: that touch is a source of comfort, security, and pleasure.

As you become more comfortable with touch, you may enjoy inventing new exercises to expand on these healthy feelings. Remember to emphasize safety, nonpressured exploring, and graduated success. Let these be your guides as you continue your journey in healthy sexuality.

- With your partner, make a plan for working on nongenital touch. You might first want to gather more resources for these activities.

- Perhaps you'll decide to work on each level of touch for a week or two.

- Be flexible. You might find some activities and levels of touch will go easily and comfortably, while others take more time. You may particularly enjoy certain ones and decide to stay at that point for a while.

- Move at a rate that feels comfortable, choosing activities that feel right for both of you. Enjoy yourselves!

IN YOUR JOURNAL

Begin each morning by writing your "daily pages." Since this chapter focuses on nongenital sex, include thoughts and discoveries about this topic in your journal.

A CLOSING EXERCISE

The closing exercise asks you and your partner to evaluate yourselves and one another. Remember, this exercise offers a wonderful opportunity for you to discover your strengths and weaknesses, as well as a chance for you and your partner to compare your perceptions of yourselves and one another.

In addition to filling out the rating scales, it will be helpful to do the following:
- Once you have filled out your scales, share the results with your fair witnesses.
- After your partner has finished, talk about your partner's perceptions too. They may differ from yours.
- If significant discrepancies exist, note them and then return to your fair witnesses to look into them more carefully.

As you work on these scales, try not to become defensive if your partner's perceptions of you differ from your own perceptions of yourself. Let these differences—and the reasons for them—be a source of information for both of you.

Part 1: Focus on You

On the first scale, consider nongenital sex as it applies to you. How comfortable are you with spending time in nongenital sexual activities? Do you rush to genital sex and orgasm? Do you talk during sex? How much work do you need on nongenital sex to feel comfortable with your skills?

Using a circle, rate yourself on the scale. (1 = low skills, need much work; 10 = high skills, need no further work.)

Next, ask your partner to rate your skills and attitude in the area of nongenital sex. Have your partner use a square to rate you.

1	2	3	4	5	6	7	8	9	10

Part 2: Focus on Your Partner

On this second scale, ask your partner to consider his or her skills and ability in the area of nongenital sex. How comfortable is your partner with spending time in nongenital sexual activities? Does your partner rush to genital sex and orgasm? Does your partner talk during sex? How much work does your partner need on nongenital sex to feel comfortable with this activity?

Have your partner use a circle to rate himself or herself.

Next, you rate your partner's skills and attitude. Use a square to do so.

1	2	3	4	5	6	7	8	9	10

Nurturing—
We learn to trust and to open our lives to experience.

Sensuality—
Through our senses, we interact with the world around us
and become connected to it.

Self-Image—
We learn that we are good and lovable.

Self-Definition—
We develop a relationship with ourselves and come to trust
ourselves. We are trustworthy.

Comfort—
We learn that we can trust others.

Knowledge—
With the acceptance of ourselves and others, we seek to grow
as people.

Relationships—
Based on what we have learned, we make the leap of trying to
live in new ways.

Partners—
We take responsibility for ourselves.

Amends—
We do what we can to correct our mistakes and improve our
lives

15

GENITAL SEX

THIS CHAPTER MAKES A KEY ASSUMPTION: Genital sex is but one dimension and one part of our sexual selves. It does, however, bring together many key issues we've examined thus far—learning to let go, nurturing, sensuality, feeling good about ourselves, knowing and trusting ourselves, knowledge of sexuality, and the ability to give ourselves over to our sensuality and sexuality. All of this comes into play at the moment of orgasm. And at that moment—the moment of *la petite mort*—we give ourselves over to a passion and a process created with our partner and culminating in the orgasm. We must surrender ourselves to the process and rely on our bodies and our partner to carry us through.

Many of the issues we work on in general in our lives—control, trust, dependency—arise during sex too. If we have trouble with trust or giving up control or surrendering, for example, our orgasm will be less than what we hope for or expect. Conversely, whenever we work on such issues in our families or in therapy, we're really contributing to healthier and more meaningful sexuality.

Thus orgasm brings into play many of the most important issues with which we deal in our lives. For the sexual anorexic, the key issues of fear and control, which lie at the core of the obsessive life, must be previously confronted to avoid problems with orgasm. Barring physical problems, most difficulties we have with orgasm find their root not in the physical, but in the mental, emotional, and spiritual dimensions of ourselves. Our difficulties are about who we are and how we feel about ourselves, and not about genitals. Knowing about sexual positions and understanding ways to improve our lovemaking are, of course, still important, but they are not as essential as knowing ourselves well.

Many men, for example, still assume that the missionary position (with the man on top and the woman underneath him) is the best way to have sex. For many women, however, this is simply not true; other positions bring greater penetration and pleasure. This reality challenges conventional male wisdom. Can the male partner be comfortable enough with who he is to accept his partner's request to do something different than what he'd been taught was best and "right"? If he's not comfortable with his identity, a simple request such as his partner asking to be on the top can cause problems for a couple. Knowing and trying different techniques is important and fun. There's excitement in variety. But of greater importance is our ability to connect with ourselves and our partner.

Making orgasm work well takes time—as anyone who's engaged in frequent anonymous sex and one-night stands would be able to tell us. Connecting with the physiology of a new person takes practice, and initial intercourse isn't always so successful because there's so much to learn about one another's body. It simply takes time to build up the awareness and communication needed for the trust that creates real passion—and, ultimately, orgasm.

In a sense, what is happening now parallels Step Ten, which says that we practice the principles we're learning in all of our relationships. To discover and live a healthy sexual life, we must practice each of the principles we've dealt with in the previous chapters. Letting go; nurturing; trusting self and others; learning to connect with ourselves, others, and the world around us; taking responsibility for our lives and relationships; making amends; repairing our relationships—all these principles are what make a healthy relationship work. We have now reached a culmination point in our emotional and spiritual growth, just as we reach the culmination of sex in orgasm. When all these principles are in place, our relationships are healed and sex can work wonderfully for us and our partner.

KEY QUESTIONS

In workshops and in my counseling experience, the following questions are often asked when we talk about genital sex.

I can do everything up to intercourse, but then I freeze. Why?

Here it is important to go back to the sexual response cycle discussed earlier and pay attention to the points in the cycle where we shut down. We need to identify what seems to be connected with this problem. It may have to do with the final "giving over" of orgasm, so we should look at what happened in the past that may be connected to this situation.

I can have an orgasm in only one very awkward and strange way. What can I do?

This is an example of what I call "hardening of the categories." Many people grew up with "rules" that told them sex only works in a particular way. Or perhaps they developed patterns around sex or achieving orgasm when they were younger, and now believe that they can't break out of them.

We do, in fact, have options with our sexuality, and part of the solution has to do with working with fantasy and acclimatizing ourselves to new ideas. We need to begin slowly, but try something different. The more options we have for pleasure, the more successful we will be. We need to remember, though, not to put too much pressure on ourselves. Change takes time.

I feel loving and want to try varied positions. My partner is not interested. In fact, he seems rigid about it and avoids me. What do I do?
This concern has more to do with the status of your relationship than with your sexuality. Perhaps, too, your partner is struggling with sexual anorexia, not you. Many factors can play a role here, and seeking counsel from a professional can help.

ISSUES

Many sexual anorexics struggle with the following issues in reference to genital sex. These issues have been explored at greater length in this or previous chapters. Read the issues carefully, noting the ones that apply to you. Then use those issues as discussion points with your partner and/or fair witnesses.

🏵 Facing problems of control and power.

🏵 Confronting impotence and preorgasmic conditions.

🏵 Isolating because of fear of inadequate performance.

🏵 Overcoming deprivation rules about pleasure.

🏵 Having irrational reactions to genitalia.

🏵 Experiencing intercourse as a loss of self.

Genital Sex

TASKS

Intercourse and orgasm touch some of our most basic control and dependency issues. These same issues are at the core of anorexic obsessions. By facing our fears about genital sex, we confront powerlessness and surrender. Orgasm may be one of the most concrete ways to encounter those fundamental life issues. Knowing positions and techniques are important for successful sex, but knowing ourselves is essential. At this point, all our issues come together at once. As we begin to explore genital life, we must remember that it is, in a way, an expression of all the other pieces of our lives.

Genital Sex—Masturbation

In talking about genital sex, perhaps it's most appropriate to start with the type of genital sex with which most people have their first experience: masturbation. Masturbation is a normal and necessary part of psychosexual development. It's a way to begin learning about our own physiology, and this makes it an indispensable part of the human sexual experience. Additionally, masturbation provides a way for us to learn what is, in fact, pleasurable so that in the future, we can communicate this information to a partner.

If we have been abused sexually, or for some other reason struggle with our sexuality, masturbation can also be an important guide or key for exploring what works sexually for us and what doesn't, as well as what for us is healthy—and unhealthy—sex. It can also provide a way to discover and remove blocks in our sexual response cycle.

Masturbation can be an important issue to examine for sex addicts too. Masturbation is sometimes problematic for them because it may have been a way to isolate themselves, and to create harmful or self-destructive fantasies. During the healing process, sex addicts may find it wise to avoid masturbation as a way to keep from going down old, familiar pathways. As an alternative, sex addicts may decide to masturbate with their partner. To masturbate with a partner in a loving relationship using healthy fantasies provides a much different and healthier experience. Sexual anorexics often find masturbation to be an excellent way to begin being sexual again.

Listen to the words of a recovering male who has been in Sex Addicts Anonymous for nearly four years now.

> When I choose to be sexual when alone, I act sexually in two ways which feel healthy for me, and which are the result of much consultation with my sponsor and group friends. For both of these, I center myself by reviewing my boundaries. I make the conscious choice to be sexual.
>
> 1. A Monogamy Fantasy: I fantasize about a single partner whom I once cared for. In this way, I do not deny my heterosexuality. With monogamy fantasy, I focus on an image of being sexual with a mate in a loving way.
> 2. Sensation Masturbation: This involves touching myself in a way which feels pleasurable. I continually ask myself and answer myself, "How does this feel?" I orient myself to my sensations instead of to addictive fetishes. I believe that in the past, I escaped personal sexual intimacy by using fantasy, which kept the focus outside myself. Now I orient to me; sex is within me. I overcome initial squeamishness of touching myself by facing my fears, not by orienting to external objects.
>
> After being sexual in a healthy way, I feel connected, proud, satisfied, warm, safe, content, and thankful.

Masturbation has long been a taboo topic in our culture and even thought to be physically harmful despite the fact that it's part of sexuality for most of us. Most sexologists now agree that masturbation is neither physically nor emotionally harmful. Many say that the pleasure, physical movement, and stress reduction gained from masturbation offer health benefits.

The following exercises are designed to help you break through some of the barriers to understanding masturbation and its role in sex, and to help you become more comfortable with this part of your sexuality.

YOU AND MASTURBATION

Write your answers to the following questions in your journal. Share your answers with your partner—or answer the questions together.

1. When you were growing up, what messages were you told about masturbation? Was it good or evil? What were you told would happen to you if you masturbated?

2. Think back to your early experiences with masturbation. How did you learn about it? What was your first time like? Were you ever caught masturbating—and, if so, what happened? We all have such stories—and here's a chance to think back on yours!

3. What did masturbation teach you about your sensuality? What did you learn about your body? About achieving orgasm? About sexual pleasure?

4. Do you still masturbate? How frequently? In what type of setting? What mental images/fantasies do you experience when you masturbate?

5. Why do you masturbate?

GENITAL PLEASURING

This exercise[1] is designed to help you discover pleasurable ways to touch your genital area. Begin by experimenting with different types of touch to your genital area. Use a personal lubricant to create new types of sensation and make genital touch easier. Try circular movements, stroking, light and hard touches. Breathe consciously. Pay attention to the way you feel. Stay present and mentally relaxed. Gradually shift from experimenting with touch to touching yourself in ways that increase pleasurable sensations. End each session with a gentle "hand hug" to your genital area.

MUTUAL MASTURBATION

At some point in our sexual lives, we may feel comfortable enough with our partner to masturbate together. Watching or being with your partner as masturbation occurs offers a wealth of information to both of you—even if you have been partners for some time. Both of you can learn more about what feels good to one another—and it can be extremely arousing for one partner to watch the other too.

The following exercises are designed to help you break through some of the barriers to understanding mutual masturbation and its role in sex, and to help you become more comfortable with this part of your sexuality.

GENITAL PLEASURING WITH A PARTNER

This exercise[2] is designed to help you explore genital touch and pleasuring. Begin by taking a shower or warm bath together. Next, do the body massage exercise described in chapter 14, but include breasts and genitals in your exploratory touch. As you begin, decide which role each of you will take—either you touching your partner's genital area or your partner touching yours.

When you are in the role of being touched, place your hand gently over your partner's hand for a while, directing your partner in the places and style you like to be touched. Communicate with your partner often. Indicate which touches you like best. Stop at any time. You may want to end with your hand resting over your partner's hand as your partner's hand hugs your genital area.

When you are in the role of touching your partner's genital area, feel free to ask your partner questions as you touch: "Does this feel good? How hard can I press here before it would be uncomfortable? What does it feel like when I pull at the skin here? Touch only as much as you feel comfortable touching in any given session.

Masturbation with a Partner

Write your answers to the following questions in your journal. When you finish, share your answers with your partner—or do the questions together.

1. When did you first masturbate with someone else, and what feelings did you experience the first time you did so?

2. What is mutual masturbation like for you now? Do you feel comfortable with doing this? Does your partner?

3. How does it feel to have your partner look at your genitals and vice versa?

4. What else do you and your partner learn about giving one another pleasure?

Sexual Intercourse

Sexual intercourse is one of the most intimate acts we can share with another person. It's more than just an exploration of one another's genitals. With intercourse we reach a deeper level of knowledge about our sexuality.

The following exercise is designed to help you break through some of the barriers to understanding sexual intercourse, and to help you become more comfortable with this part of your sexuality.

You and Intercourse

Write your answers to the following questions in your journal. When you finish, share your answers with your partner.

1. What positions have you and your partner used when making love? Are you both satisfied with what you know about sexual positions? If you want to know more, seek out information about various intercourse positions and try the ones that seem intriguing and appealing.

2. Where do you and your partner have intercourse? Are there places you've fantasized about having intercourse, but haven't? What about your partner?

3. Can you think of any scenarios in which you'd like to have intercourse that would be stimulating and helpful to you, but have not? What are they?

4. What does it feel like when you have intercourse with your partner? What does it feel like when you're inside one another?

5. When you are having intercourse, what thoughts do you have—about the experience, about your partner, and so on—that you want to tell your partner but have not?

6. What inhibitions do you experience during intercourse?

After trying new positions and talking about sex, we still return to the fundamental reality that for all of this to work, we must feel good about ourselves and about accepting pleasure. All the principles we've talked about thus far must be looked at before healthy sex can take place.

Try not to expect anything from sex—expectation thwarts so much. Relax, enjoy one another, and let things happen as they will. Remember, too, that there are times in any relationship when partners are at odds with one another. In addition, many men will struggle with impotence as they age, and many women will have times during menopause when sex is the last thing on their minds. Keep in mind that the genitals are not the main sex organ of the body—it's the mind.

PLANNING

The exercises in this chapter asked you to think about your sexuality in the areas of masturbation, mutual masturbation, and sexual intercourse. These exercises asked you not only to look at your sexual history and attitudes, but also to try new activities and ideas.

- Look back through those exercises and decide on additional activities you would like to bring into your sex life.

- Next, make a plan or schedule as to roughly when you will try these activities. Perhaps, for example, you'll decide to experiment more with mutual masturbation over a period of three or four weeks and, during the same time, try three or four new positions for intercourse.

Whatever you decide to do is fine, but making a plan and drawing up a rough schedule will help you follow through on your goals.

IN YOUR JOURNAL

Start each morning by writing your "daily pages." Since this chapter focuses on genital sex, include thoughts and discoveries about this topic in your journal.

A CLOSING EXERCISE

✐ The closing exercise asks you and your partner to evaluate yourselves and one another. Remember, this exercise offers a wonderful opportunity for you to discover your strengths and weaknesses, as well as a chance for you and your partner to compare your perceptions of yourselves and one another.

In addition to filling out the rating scales, it will be helpful to do the following:

- Once you have filled out your scales, share the results with your fair witnesses.
- After your partner has finished, talk about your partner's perceptions too. They may differ from yours.
- If significant discrepancies exist, note them and then return to your fair witnesses to look into them more carefully.

As you work on these scales, try not to become defensive if your partner's perceptions differ from your own perceptions of yourself. Let these differences—and the reasons for them—be a source of information for both of you.

Part 1: Focus on You

On the first scale, consider genital sex as it applies to you. How comfortable are you with genital sexual activities? Do you feel blocked in any part of the sexual response cycle? Are you able to incorporate new activities to enhance your mutual pleasure? How much work do you need on genital sex to feel comfortable?

Using a circle, rate yourself on the scale. (1 = low skills, need much work; 10 = high skills, need no further work.)

Next, ask your partner to rate you. Have your partner use a square.

I   2   3   4   5   6   7   8   9   10

Part 2: Focus on Your Partner

On this second scale, ask your partner to consider his or her skills and ability in the area of genital sex. How comfortable is your partner with genital sexual activities? Does your partner feel blocked in any part of the sexual response cycle? Is your partner able to incorporate new activities to enhance your mutual pleasure? How much work does your partner need on genital sex to feel comfortable?

Have your partner use a circle to rate himself or herself.

Next, you rate your partner's skills and ability. Use a square to do so.

I   2   3   4   5   6   7   8   9   10

Nurturing—
We learn to trust and to open our lives to experience.

Sensuality—
Through our senses, we interact with the world around us
and become connected to it.

Self-Image—
We learn that we are good and lovable.

Self-Definition—
We develop a relationship with ourselves and come to trust
ourselves. We are trustworthy.

Comfort—
We learn that we can trust others.

Knowledge—
With the acceptance of ourselves and others, we seek to grow
as people.

Relationships—
Based on what we have learned, we make the leap of trying to
live in new ways.

Partners—
We take responsibility for ourselves.

Amends—
We do what we can to correct our mistakes and improve our
lives.

Living our values—
We practice these principles in all parts of our lives.

16

SPIRITUALITY

I distrust any religious conversion which does not also involve an intensification of one's sexuality.

—M. Scott Peck

The Road Less Traveled

TOO OFTEN IN OUR CULTURE, we see the relationship of sexuality and spirituality as a war in which one must defeat and destroy the other. This is, however, futile. The desire to unite through the sexual act can metaphorically be seen as a drive to once again be united with the Divine. This is a yearning for our lost wholeness, a search for our other half that we might, if even for only a moment through sexual union, reexperience the lost bliss of our Godlike totality. Our sexuality arises out of a sense of incompleteness that is manifested by an urge toward wholeness and a yearning for the Godhead.

But what, then, is spirituality? Is it not this same desire, arising out of a sense of incompleteness and manifested in an urge toward wholeness and a yearning for the Divine? While spirituality and sexuality are not exactly the same, they are cut from the same cloth. They are, as Scott Peck says, "kissing cousins." The sexual and spiritual parts of our being lie so close together that it is hardly possible to arouse one without arousing the other. To me, sexuality and spirituality are like two snare drums sitting side by side. If you strike one, the other vibrates too.

This is not myth; it's human experience. In Peck's *The Road Less Traveled*, he writes, "When my beloved first stands before me naked, all open to my sight, there is a feeling throughout the whole of me. Awe! Why Awe? If sex is no more than an instinct, why don't I simply feel horny or hungry? Such simple hunger would be quite sufficient to ensure the propagation of the species. Why should sex be complicated with reverence?"

Sex is "complicated with reverence" because it is, in fact, the closest many people ever come to a mystical experience. Indeed, this is why so many people chase after sex with such desperate abandon. Whether or not they know it, they are searching for God.

In his studies, Abraham Maslow discovered that self-actualizing people often experience orgasm as a religious, even mystical, event. Maslow makes it clear that these people were not speaking metaphorically. With another human in deeply loving relationships, we can touch the Divine through sex. Ironically, however, though we need the other person to reach these heights, we briefly lose that person at the climactic moment, forgetting who and where we are. Mystics and spiritual teachers through the ages have spoken of an "ego death" as a necessary part of the spiritual journey—even its goal— and the French, as previously pointed out, refer to orgasm as "the little death." We have entered the realm of spirit. Sex and spirit become one as we become one with All.

Sex does, however, complicate relationships. It is the search for God in human romantic relationships that lies at the root of the problem, says Peck. We look to our spouse or to romantic love to meet all our needs and fulfill us. This never works, at least not for long. We can live in the bliss of new love perhaps for a few months, a year, or even a few years if we are lucky. But after a while, we change or our partner changes or everything changes—and suddenly it's all up for grabs.

Throughout this long journey, however, we learn a lot about vulnerability and intimacy and love and whittling away at our narcissism. It is natural for us humans to want a tangible God, but the Divine is not ours to possess. Instead, we must learn to accept that we live within the Divine—or, as some Native American cultures describe it, The One in Whom We Live and Move and Have Our Being.

The common denominator of sex and spirituality is the search for meaning. Sexuality and spirituality connect through meaning. As we deepen our understanding of ourselves, of others, of our planet and all its myriad life, we heighten both our spirituality and our sexuality. As Peck is fond of saying, "I distrust any religious conversion which does not also involve an intensification of one's sexuality." The deeper and more meaningful our sexuality, the more we touch the mystical.

We need to recognize that we are part of a much larger whole, and it's when people are unable to make this connection that they turn to relationships with objects—the false gods, in the biblical sense, of alcohol, money, sex, food—whatever seems to fill the void inside. While still a search for meaning, this path leads to addiction and a life unmanageable, out of control.

Here is a critically important point. The choice is not to be in control or out of control; the choice is how we will live without control. Either we "lose" control by admitting that larger forces are at work in our lives and that we are part of a Divine plan or we lose control by succumbing to compulsive and addictive behaviors. The former brings us closer to our true selves and the Divine; the latter brings pain, misery, and, ultimately, self-destruction.

These ideas parallel the sense of the Eleventh Step, which says that through prayer and meditation, we seek conscious contact with a Higher Power—a connection that we strengthen as we learn to accept nurturing, to be open to our senses, to trust ourselves and others, and to become more centered within ourselves. As we do this, we are better able to enter into healthy relationships with a partner. Our search for meaning weaves the strands of relationship, self, spirit, and sensuality/sexuality together.

Let me tell you a personal story that illustrates these ideas. It takes place when I was in first grade. I was raised Catholic, and right before Christmas that year, the priest in our little country parish called my mother and asked if I could serve as an altar boy on Christmas morning. I expressed some fear, because I had never done this before, nor had I been through the "altar boy training program." Father Yanny told me to come early Christmas morning and he would show me what I needed to do.

On that fateful morning, I dutifully showed up early at the church. My mother, thrilled at the prospect of my serving at mass on Christmas morning, had invited her five sisters and their families to join us. This had now become a high-drama event, and I was getting more nervous by the minute. Old Father Yanny, however, was very reassuring. There were only two things I had to remember, he said. One was when to move the "Book" from one side of the altar to the other, and the second was to ring a set of bells whenever he put his right hand on the altar. In those days, the bell signaled the congregation to kneel, sit, or stand at different points in the liturgy.

Father Yanny was getting on in years, and he probably wasn't aware that he often leaned on the altar to steady himself—using his right hand. Mass began, and when Father Yanny leaned, I rang. When I rang, the congregation moved. I had that church going up and down, up and down. My mother was mortified, but my aunts thought it was great, and they tell the story to this day.

As I look back on this event, what really strikes me now as an adult is that those people in that church knew the bells were being rung at the wrong time. And they knew exactly when to stand, sit, or kneel without the help of the bells. But they followed them, thus going through motions no longer attached to the meaning of the service. I think of that experience as a metaphor for religion as many people see it today—forced motions detached from any deeper meaning. How many of us have become separated from our spiritual lives because the rituals of religion no longer fit our lives?

For sexual anorexics and the sex addicts, sex has been devoid of meaning and the source of tremendous loneliness and suffering. I remember one patient who told this story about family week at an addictions treatment center. It was Sunday morning and his spouse was attending services in a church across the road from the center. He sat in his room, looking at that church, knowing that she was inside. He was moved by her faithfulness to him, especially about how important their relationship was to her. With that emotion, he had a flash of insight about how putting "faith" in the wrong things was a major part of his illness. With the tears that came, he felt connected to his wife and to the presence of his Higher Power. For many of us, the story is the same. Spiritual connection happens when we admit suffering. Acknowledging our suffering, and what we learn from it in our life journey, is of incredible importance. As we change our lives by working on our problems, we connect what's meaningful in our lives with our spirituality. And sex in the context of a meaningful relationship with ourselves and another can become an opportunity to go far beyond the simple physiology of being sexual—it becomes part of our spiritual expression.

Expressing the Spirituality of Sex

One of the troubles that couples have, in addition to communicating in general about sex, is talking about what is meaningful or spiritual during sex. It is relatively easy to share spiritual feelings in a worship community. It's easy to acknowledge and express our spirituality to ourselves. But to express our spirituality to a partner who knows us well is one of the greatest challenges we have. Why? Because in a group there is a kind of anonymity, and there is anonymity when we're alone. To share a spiritual moment with someone with whom we are deeply involved makes us tremendously vulnerable and it can be truly frightening.

If, then, we add to this situation attempts to communicate about our sexuality, with the risk and vulnerability that entails, we have perhaps one of the most vulnerable moments that a couple can experience. To be able to tell your partner at the very moment during sex that something important to you is happening, and to tell just how significant or spiritual that moment is, is difficult and awkward, and requires taking a great risk. It is one of the greatest challenges we have as human beings. But to take that risk and speak about the moment makes it all the more extraordinary and precious.

How, then, can we change this situation, particularly in a culture in which it's so unusual for people to talk about what's truly meaningful to them? Let me make three suggestions. First, we need to discover what moves us when we're sexual. What gives sex meaning for us? I remember, for example, the night my daughter Erin was conceived. Today, I'm no longer married to Erin's mother, but that in no way diminishes the importance or significance of what happened that night.

Secondly, we need to look back in our lives and search out the moments that were sexually significant for us. As we do, a pattern about what has value for us will emerge.

Finally, we can begin talking with others about these matters. If something happens that we really value, we need to let our partner know—when it's happening. Don't wait. We need to stop and say, "I really like this" or "What we did just now was so special for me." In addition, as previously noted, we need to talk about our sexuality with others besides our partner. Sex isn't something shameful or dirty that needs to be kept from our friends or families. We need to be more open. As we speak out, we remove sex from the hidden, secret place we, in this culture, have kept it for so long. Much of the sexual pathology in our culture—child abuse, sex offenses, and so on—happen within the context of secrecy. They are in the dark side. We must break the no-talk rule if for no other reason than that sex is too significant a part of our spiritual lives to hide.

Let me close with a statement written by a fellow I met some years ago. It is to me a wonderful and simple expression of the spirituality of sex.

> Healthy sexual behavior for me includes savoring moments. When I was thirteen years old and involved in my first steady relationship, there was one particular night which for me exemplified healthy sexuality. That night, I was walking my girl-friend home in the rain on a warm night. On the way, we stopped in the road, under a streetlight. There we kissed and held each other as the rain beat down harder upon us. There was something sweet, majestic, and natural in what happened that night. I felt connected, valued, and physically alive. The thought of that night brings enchanted memories and hope to me. That experience was very sexual, healing, innocent, and nongenital.
>
> It took a spiritual leap for me to begin enjoying sex again—either alone or in a relationship. With surprise, I found foreplay can be exciting, enjoying my body's sensation, savoring orgasm in the knowledge that despair will not result.

KEY QUESTIONS

Typically in workshops and in my counseling experience, the following questions are asked when we talk about becoming more spiritual.

*Sex is natural and fun, so why do people have to make it
into this big deal? Why is it not enough to have a good
relationship and satisfying sex?*

Why make this thing into a big deal? Too often, we push
aside the deeper feelings that arise during sex as a way to
avoid the intimacy that sustains an enduring relationship.
We cannot have shared common experiences that include
our sexuality without sooner or later acknowledging these
deeper realities. Intimacy demands that we talk about our
lives together. Indeed, to have intimacy is to talk about our
lives together.

Why is sex so boring sometimes?

Sex can be boring for us because we don't have the level of
honesty (we've discussed this earlier) that can bring ongoing renewal to our relationship. We don't need to be constantly spontaneous or developing new fantasies, though as
we've seen, they do add freshness to our relationship. Sex
will continue to be interesting and exciting and new if we
simply acknowledge the deeper parts of our sexual reality.

ISSUES

Many sexual anorexics struggle with the following issues in
reference to spirituality. Some of these issues have been
explored at greater length in this or previous chapters; for
those that have not, a brief discussion is included here. Read
the issues carefully, noting the ones that apply to you. Then
use those issues as discussion points with your partner and/or
fair witnesses.

❀ Failing to operate on a basis of meaning.

When we lose ourselves as anorexics lose themselves or as
addicts lose themselves, we are no longer living with a conscious
connection between ourselves and the Divine. As a result, we

experience separation, rather than having our actions flow out into the world from a deeply felt spiritual core.

❊ Being unable to express what is valuable or important.
This is characteristic of failing to operate from a basis of meaning. Most of us—particularly if we have a history of family or relationship dysfunction or abuse—find it difficult to talk about what we find important or valuable. We feel that by so doing, we open ourselves to ridicule or rejection or, at the very least, we feel that we'll not be taken seriously. To express what we really need and value is simply one of the hardest things any of us can do.

❊ Being comfortable with a double life in which important things do not get discussed or shared.
This is one of the common issues. It means, for example, that the addict and anorexic pretend to be something they are not. On the surface, a sex addict may appear to be living faithfully, but scratch through that veneer and we'll find he's maintaining a secret life. A sexual anorexic may be sexual and appear to her partner to be enjoying intercourse immensely, but in reality, she is terrified of sex. That enjoyment is only an act. Both the addict and the anorexic are leading double lives, and both have fundamental incongruities in their lives—lives marked by a host of dishonesties.

❊ Having difficulty with accountability and commitment because of fear of being counted or taking a stand.
This is where being who you are and living up to what you say your mission is becomes very important. If you can't do that, it's very difficult to be held accountable or make a commitment.

❊ Having no models for communicating or creating meaning.
Many of us have come from families in which we had no example of either of these skills. No one showed us how to communicate or create meaning.

TASKS

Even pornography can teach us about genital functioning. Movies and novels can teach us about romance. Where, however, can a couple learn about communicating meaning concurrently and consistently, especially when dysfunction has been the model for meaning? Sex is about meaning. Life change is about meaning. Both have a spiritual base. And sexual change is forged in the depths of personal suffering and tempered with play, nurturing, and trust. These can provide new paths to sexual meaning and spirituality.

Your Sexuality and Spirituality

An exercise in an earlier chapter asked you about your sexual history. This exercise asks for something a bit different. Think of the times in your life when sex truly moved you in a meaningful and spiritual way, a way that had great value or significance or that helped you feel more connected to the universe and your Higher Power. An example from my life would be the conception of my children. In your journal, list those special times, and then briefly explain why each was meaningful.

1. Now that you have completed your list, study it and try to see what these moments have in common.

2. What did you discover about yourself and your sexuality by doing this exercise?

Contact Portrait

This exercise asks you and your partner to create what's known as a "contact portrait." Here are your directions:
• Choose a time when you will not be interrupted—and a place in which you both find it easy to be comfortable. You'll need to have a large piece of newsprint and some crayons or magic markers too.

• Put the piece of paper between you. Your challenge is to have a conversation about what is meaningful about your relationship for fifteen to thirty minutes—WITHOUT TALKING! You may communicate only by drawing pictures and symbols on the piece of paper between you—the alphabet is off-limits too!

• When you're finished, talk (yes, words are acceptable now!) about what you were trying to say to each another. As you will see, this is an exercise in communication as well as an opportunity to learn more about your relationship.

PLANNING

Make a plan covering the next two to four weeks. Decide how and when you will take time to do the above exercises and to talk with one another about them. Using ideas discussed in this chapter, try to make this communication part of your sexual experience too.

IN YOUR JOURNAL

Start each morning by writing your "daily pages." In addition, since this chapter focuses on spirituality, your writing should focus on spirituality as well. What gives your life meaning? What has most moved you during sex? In your own words, how can sex be spiritual?

A CLOSING EXERCISE

The closing exercise asks you and your partner to evaluate yourselves and one another. Remember, this exercise offers a wonderful opportunity for you to discover your strengths and weaknesses, as well as a chance for you and your partner to compare your perceptions of yourselves and one another.

In addition to filling out the rating scales, it will be helpful to do the following:
- Once you have filled out your scales, share the results with your fair witnesses.
- After your partner has finished, talk about your partner's perceptions too. They may differ from yours and/or those of your fair witnesses.
- If significant discrepancies exist, note them and then return to your fair witnesses to look into them more carefully.

As you work on these scales, try not to become defensive if the perceptions your partner or your fair witnesses have of you differ from your own perceptions of yourself. Let these differences—and the reasons for them—be a source of information for all of you.

If you are not currently in a relationship, ask one of your fair witnesses (therapist, sponsor, anorexia group member, Twelve Step support group member, or RCA group member, for example) to work through the scales with you.

Part 1: Focus on You

Consider spirituality as it relates to your sexuality. Can you accept sex as a spiritual act? Are you aware of meaningful spiritual moments during sex? Can you express such moments with your partner? Do you try to "stay connected" with your higher self during sex? How much work do you need in this area?

Using a circle, rate yourself on the scale below. (1 = low skills, need much work; 10 = high skills, need no further work.)

Next, ask your partner to rate your sexuality and spirituality. Have your partner use a square to rate you.

| 1 | 2 | 3 | 4 | 5 | 6 | 7 | 8 | 9 | 10 |

Spirituality

Part 2: Focus on Your Partner

On this second scale, ask your partner to consider spirituality as it applies to him or her. Can your partner accept sex as a spiritual act? Is your partner aware of meaningful spiritual moments during sex? Can your partner express such moments with you? Does your partner try to "stay connected" during sex?

Have your partner use a circle to rate himself or herself.

Next, you rate your partner's spirituality as it applies to sexuality. Use a square to do so.

I   2   3   4   5   6   7   8   9   10

Nurturing—
We learn to trust and to open our lives to experience.

Sensuality—
Through our senses, we interact with the world around us
and become connected to it.

Self-Image—
We learn that we are good and lovable.

Self-Definition—
We develop a relationship with ourselves and come to trust
ourselves. We are trustworthy.

Comfort—
We learn that we can trust others.

Knowledge—
With the acceptance of ourselves and others, we seek to grow
as people.

Relationships—
Based on what we have learned, we make the leap of trying to
live in new ways.

Partners—
We take responsibility for ourselves.

Amends—
We do what we can to correct our mistakes and improve our
lives.

Living our values—
We practice these principles in all parts of our lives.

Spirituality—
Living our principles leads to a deep spiritual connectedness.

17

PASSION

Nothing is of value to you unless you are willing to publicly declare it.

—Sidney Simon
Values Clarification

THROUGHOUT THIS BOOK I have stressed the great importance of discovering what in our lives is truly meaningful to us and then ensuring that these values are linked to our sexuality. More than thirty years ago, author Sidney Simon created a valuable series of achievement and personal growth exercises for teachers and children to use in school. He published these exercises in a book entitled *Values Clarification*.

In this book, Simon made a statement that moved me deeply when I first read it, and I still believe it has profound implications for all of us. He says, "Nothing is of value to you unless you are willing to publicly declare it." In other words, if we publicly declare a belief and take action based on that belief, or behave in a way appropriate to that belief, then we can truly say it is a value for us. Conversely, to say we hold a belief, but remain unwilling to publicly state it or own it or defend it, means that this belief is not a value.

This idea of *publicly* declaring or passing on what we have learned and believe is a critical ingredient in the success of

Twelve Step programs. The Twelfth Step, in fact, states, "Having had a spiritual awakening as the result of these steps, we tried to carry this message to [others], and to practice these principles in all our affairs." This idea has been present from the very beginnings of Alcoholics Anonymous (AA) when Carl Jung, the famous psychologist and writer, in correspondence with Bill W., founder along with Dr. Bob of AA, stated that alcoholics would never be able to stay sober unless they were able to witness to others and pass on their stories.

Trying to carry out Jung's suggestions on how to stay sober, Bill W. and Dr. Bob went to Akron General Hospital in Akron, Ohio, to visit a man who would become the third member of AA. As the story is told, this man had been in and out of hospitals for years trying to stay sober, but despite all this professional help, he'd been unable to quit drinking. He was about to be released after having been detoxified yet one more time when Dr. Bob and Bill W. came up to his wife, who was standing outside his hospital room, and said, "We're alcoholics. We're drunks. We need to talk to your husband in order for us to stay sober."

She wasn't quite sure what to make of their request; but, nevertheless, she went in and said to her husband, "You know, there are a couple drunks outside who say they need your help." He told his wife that he wasn't the sort of person who would refuse someone in need, and, of course, he'd just have to give them the wisdom of his many years of experience. So he, Bill W., and Dr. Bob told their stories to one another, and through sharing their stories, the man realized how much he was like his visitors. Together, these three men went on to help build AA. Tremendous wisdom can be carried in a sharing of one's experience.

The Power of Stories

As therapists have long known, stories can be far more effective than simple logic in helping people accept solutions to their problems. Eric Erickson, the famous therapist, often said that when he had a particularly difficult patient, he would eventually pause and say, "You know, I knew someone like you once." Erickson would then spin out a story that carried the lesson he was trying to convey. By the end of the story, a solution would appear with which the patient could identify.

The sharing of *our* stories is a key part of the strength and wisdom of Twelve Step programs—and such public declarations contain an important lesson. If we have found something that gives our lives meaning and we feel this deeply, then we need to take the next step. We must be willing to tell others about our experiences, and we must act on our beliefs, thus living our values.

When a person has had a life-changing experience, and then gives witness to it, the power of such actions can move others to change and grow. How, you might ask, can that happen? Think about how we describe such "storytellers." We call them passionate. We say they are passionate about what they believe and about their experiences. And when people are passionate about their stories, we are more likely to take the story in and be changed by it.

As noted, our ability to talk about sex has been very limited in our culture. Many families create no-talk rules about sexuality. The same has long been true for public talk about sex. Today, we are barraged by talk of sex in the media, but this talk is not about meaning or values; stories of scandal and sleaze seem to be the predominant topics. The visual and auditory buzz of sexuality has little to do with our experiences of what gives our sexuality meaning.

Our Stories Have Culture-wide Impact

I wrote this book to help people who want to develop a healthier sexuality and to help professionals interested in assisting clients or colleagues to do likewise. As noted in chapter 1, we are living in a time of extraordinary change. A profound paradigm shift is taking place, one that includes a movement away from the patriarchal paradigm of sexual control, exploitation, and manipulation in which sex is a commodity, traded even within the context of partner-based relationships. The paradigm toward which we are moving includes a recognition of everyone's dignity and of the value of each gender and a respect for our differences—life marked by kindness and generosity and a nonviolent healthy sexuality. If we can move to embrace the model described in chapter 1, the implications for our culture are of extraordinary significance.

We are challenging some of the deepest premises of our culture—ones that trap us in so much turmoil and violence. Taken in this context, the changes we make in our own lives go beyond our individual recoveries. We're doing more than helping our immediate friends, family members, and colleagues. By changing our lives, we are truly acting to bring about this new paradigm—one which, as previously stated, can only emerge when our sexual attitudes change.

Thus, we need to be more clear in public about the values we hold for our sexual lives. We need to act on those values. Only then will we move from a culture obsessed with sex, one that routinely teaches us to view people as sex objects, and that refuses to openly examine its sexual attitudes. Through our actions, we will participate in and advance cultural change. This is incredibly significant work to which each of us can contribute by our willingness to face and speak out about these issues.

Gregory Bateson spoke of addiction as "prayer gone awry." Addiction is a life gone out of control in a negative direction, one in which meaning is sought in an object outside the self. We do need to "lose control," but in a spiritual sense. We need to take the leap of faith that will let us publicly move in a new direction, and then talk about it openly. Whether we are in prayer or in passion, being out of control requires the same leap. To do either, we must give up control and put ourselves at risk. We move from observing life to participating in life— and that, of course, means as a sexual person too.

Seven Levels of Feeling

To me, passion becomes the culmination of a learning journey in which we at last determine and claim our values. It's a journey that begins in childhood with our earliest feelings and proceeds through seven levels, as shown in figure 17.1.

Figure 17.1

<table>
<tr><td colspan="2" align="center">Seven Levels of Feeling</td></tr>
<tr><td>Level 1</td><td>Intuitively experiencing the world . . . and our sexuality.</td></tr>
<tr><td>Level 2</td><td>Use of language begins. New messages to cope with, including ones about sex.</td></tr>
<tr><td>Level 3</td><td>Puberty brings countless new feelings.</td></tr>
<tr><td>Level 4</td><td>Discovering the need for focus and discipline. Beginnings of understanding own limitations.</td></tr>
<tr><td>Level 5</td><td>Learning about romantic/sexual relationships, childbirth, parenting.</td></tr>
<tr><td>Level 6</td><td>Dominant threads of life and culture come together. Beginning to see interrelatednesss and sacredness of creation.</td></tr>
<tr><td>Level 7</td><td>Learning to live authentically in intimate and public/social relationships. Life becomes public declaration of who we are.</td></tr>
</table>

At the first level of feeling, we intuitively experience our sexuality. Using a term coined by therapist and trauma expert Marilyn Murray, we speak about the *original feeling child*—how we all were before we received any messages about the world.[1]

When we begin to acquire language, we move to the second level of feeling. We now have words to use, and this brings in all types of messages with which we must cope, including ones about sex. At this time, some of our early knowledge becomes obscured or is seen as stolen or forbidden.

As we begin to experience our sexuality and pass through puberty, we reach a third level of knowing and feeling. We have countless new feelings. This stage parallels, in a sense, the first because we are again enveloped by so much that is new to us. We are again close to the original voice of who we are sexually.

Part of this new experience leads us to the knowledge that we can't do everything that our feelings dictate. At the fourth level, we discover that we need to develop focus and discipline in order to allow our sexuality to work well for us. This sense of understanding our own human limitations is essentially the passage into adulthood.

As we move in and out of relationships in the fifth level, we learn more and more about what it means to be in romantic/sexual relationships. Once in a permanent relationship, we discover the joys and challenges of growing with another person. We have the experience of childbirth and parenting.

In time, we also begin to weave together the dominant threads of life and culture. In the sixth level, we begin to see the interrelatedness and sacredness of all creation.

In the seventh and final level, we begin to understand what it means to live a congruent life, one in which we are able to live authentically in both our intimate relationships and our public and social relationships. Our lives become a public declaration of who we are.

Ideally, we are able to grow through these natural stages, but, unfortunately, this process can be sidetracked much too easily, as has happened to sexual anorexics and sex addicts.

Despite such difficulties, it's so important to understand, first, that we can recover from the damage we suffered and, second, that our experiences and struggles add to the meaning in our lives and help us know what we must speak out against. I firmly believe that the very people who have suffered most are the truest and most important voices we have at this time. The abuse survivors. The sexual anorexics. The sex addicts. The codependents. All these people bring their unique points of view together to form common elements of a broader truth. In so doing, they recover the sensibilities of their original feeling child and bring all of us closer to significant cultural change. The people whom I have seen take this step have made *tremendous* contributions to themselves and to those around them.

Speaking Out and Giving Back

There are many, many ways we can support the changes toward which we are all working. In a Twelve Step program meeting, for example, recovering individuals can talk about their experiences and their recovery. Sexual anorexics and others *need* to talk about this out loud—to talk about the extreme healing that they've experienced—because this will make an enormous difference in their ability to complete the cycle. Individuals can, of course, still maintain a level of privacy, but the same energy that makes the Twelve Steps work in the first place will also help heal their sexuality.

The following are examples of additional ways we can speak our truth.

- Write a letter to the editor when we see something untoward in a newspaper.

- Speak out whenever we see discrimination in the form of sexualized rage or prejudice about any sexual issue. Don't let it go by, thinking, "Oh, that's too bad."

- Work to ensure that children are taught appropriately about sexuality, and that they can learn about it in safety.

- Work toward eradicating sexual trauma and prejudice within our governmental institutions, businesses, and churches.

- Act in ways that bring dignity to both women and men.

KEY QUESTIONS

Typically in workshops and in my counseling experience, the following questions are asked when we talk about becoming more passionate.

I'm struggling to have feelings in general, let alone sexual ones. How do I reclaim my feelings beyond arousal?
Again, this is an area for which no magic switch exists. If we're generally out of touch with our feelings, we'll find it very difficult to have sexual feelings beyond the basic physiological sexual response. Part of our recovery includes opening to our feelings. Refer again to chapters 6 and 7.

Why do I feel that if I am passionate, I will lose somehow?
Many of us grew up in families in which we were somehow penalized for being honest or real. Perhaps, for example, we were ridiculed or punished for this. Passion grows out of an honest expression of one's self; when such expression is restricted, part of the price we pay is the loss of our ability to be passionate. We can reclaim our passion by living our values and beliefs.

Passion

ISSUES

Many sexual anorexics struggle with the following issues in reference to passion. These issues have been explored at greater length in this or previous chapters. Read the issues carefully, noting the ones that apply to you. Then use those issues as discussion points with your partner and/or fair witnesses.

🌺 Feeling incongruent or unreal when passionate.

🌺 Having difficulty giving up control.

🌺 Acting in to avoid acting out.

🌺 Being solemn and grim as a way to avoid passion.

🌺 Growing up in rigid, disengaged family environments that extinguished passion.

🌺 Reclaiming feelings obliterated by obsession.

TASKS

Passion and spirituality are antidotes to obsession. This means that as individuals, we must leave the "observer-of-life" status and actively participate in the world around us—as well as embrace our sexuality.

The following exercise will help you integrate what you have learned throughout the chapters in this book. Before you begin, complete the "Before and After—Sharing Perceptions" exercises on pages 359–63. They will help you better recognize the changes you're making in your life. The final, combined scales will declare your progress and show what your sexual healing journey has been about. They are a visible record of ways that you've changed.

A DEBRIEFING

Call your fair witnesses together and talk with them about what you've learned. Describe what your journey has been like—do this orally or in written form. Tell your story. Tell what's happened to you.

1. Describe to your fair witnesses what you've been through.

2. Describe to your fair witnesses what this process means to you now.

3. State how you have changed. In what ways are you a different person now?

4. State what you are now going to do differently in your life.

5. State some of the ways you will publicly witness to your "conversion"—your new beliefs, values, and ways of living.

By telling your story to others, you make your stated values truly your own. A kind of public "ownership" about the *concrete* actions you are going to take—both to change your own life and to influence the larger culture—now exists.

IN YOUR JOURNAL

Start each morning by writing your "daily pages." In addition, since this chapter focuses on passion, create a passion inventory. What do you feel passionate about? What makes you feel passionate?

A CLOSING EXERCISE

✐ The closing exercise asks you and your partner to evaluate yourselves and one another. Remember, this exercise offers a wonderful opportunity for you to discover your strengths and weaknesses, as well as a chance for you and your partner to compare your perceptions of yourselves and one another. Over the course of chapters 6 through 17, these exercises should have helped you chart your progress in building a healthy sexuality.

In addition to filling out the rating scales, it will be helpful to do the following:

- Once you have filled out your scales, share the results with your fair witnesses.
- After your partner has finished, talk about your partner's perceptions too. They may differ from yours and/or those of your fair witnesses.
- If significant discrepancies exist, note them and then return to your fair witnesses to look into them more carefully.

As you work on the scales, try not to become defensive if the perceptions your partner or your fair witnesses have of you differ from your own perceptions of yourself. Let these differences—and the reasons for them—be a source of information for all of you.

If you are not currently in a relationship, ask one of your fair witnesses (therapist, sponsor, anorexia group member, Twelve Step support group member, or RCA group member, for example) to work through the scales with you.

Part 1: Focus on You

Consider passion as it applies to you. Are you blocking passion in your life? How passionate do you feel about your life now? Are you able to feel more passion now than before you began working through the strategies and principles in this book? Are you comfortable feeling passion?

Using a circle, rate yourself on the scale below. (1 = low skills, need much work; 10 = high skills, need no further work.)

Next, ask your partner to rate your passion. Have your partner use a square to rate you.

I   2   3   4   5   6   7   8   9   10

Part 2: Focus on Your Partner

On this second scale, ask your partner to consider passion as it applies to him or her. Is your partner blocking passion in his or her life? How passionate does your partner feel about life? Is your partner able to feel more passion now than before you both began this process? Is your partner comfortable feeling passion?

Have your partner use a circle to rate himself or herself.

Next, you rate your partner in the area of passion. Use a square to do so.

I   2   3   4   5   6   7   8   9   10

Nurturing—
We learn to trust and to open our lives to experience.

Sensuality—
Through our senses, we interact with the world around us and become connected to it.

Self-Image—
We learn that we are good and lovable.

Self-Definition—
We develop a relationship with ourselves and come to trust ourselves. We are trustworthy.

Comfort—
We learn that we can trust others.

Knowledge—
With the acceptance of ourselves and others, we seek to grow as people.

Relationships—
Based on what we have learned, we make the leap of trying to live in new ways.

Partners—
We take responsibility for ourselves.

Amends—
We do what we can to correct our mistakes and improve our lives.

Living our values—
We practice these principles in all parts of our lives.

Spirituality—
Living our principles leads to a deep spiritual connectedness.

Passion—
We witness to the world.

BEFORE AND AFTER—SHARING PERCEPTIONS

My ratings of myself, and my ratings of my partner

You'll need two pens or markers, each with a different color. Begin by rating your abilities or comfort level and those of your partner in each of the twelve categories on the combined scales below. (1 = low skills, need much work; 10 = high skills, need no further work.) These ratings should reflect how you see yourself and your partner *today* after completing this book. Use a circle to rate yourself and a square to rate your partner.

Next, go back to all the previous "Focus on You" scales, note your ratings, and use the second pen or marker to transfer them to the "master" scales below. Do the same with your partner's previous ratings. Again, use a circle for your rating and a square for your partner's.

When you finish, you will be able to see the changes you have made.

NURTURING

I   2   3   4   5   6   7   8   9   10

SENSUALITY

I   2   3   4   5   6   7   8   9   10

SELF-IMAGE

I   2   3   4   5   6   7   8   9   10

SELF-DEFINITION

I   2   3   4   5   6   7   8   9   10

COMFORT

I   2   3   4   5   6   7   8   9   10

KNOWLEDGE

I   2   3   4   5   6   7   8   9   10

RELATIONSHIP

I   2   3   4   5   6   7   8   9   10

PARTNERS

I   2   3   4   5   6   7   8   9   10

NONGENITAL SEX

I   2   3   4   5   6   7   8   9   10

GENITAL SEX

I   2   3   4   5   6   7   8   9   10

SPIRITUALITY

I   2   3   4   5   6   7   8   9   10

PASSION

I   2   3   4   5   6   7   8   9   10

BEFORE AND AFTER—SHARING PERCEPTIONS

My partner's ratings of himself or herself, and my partner's ratings of me

Again, you'll need two pens or markers with differing colors. Your partner should begin by rating his or her abilities or comfort level in each of the twelve categories on the combined scales below. (1 = low skills, need much work; 10 = high skills, need no further work.) Then have your partner rate you. These ratings should reflect how your partner sees himself or herself and you today after completing this book. Your partner should use a circle to rate himself or herself and a square to rate you.

Next, your partner should go back to all the previous "Focus on Your Partner" scales, note how he or she rated himself or herself, and use the second pen or marker to transfer the ratings to the "master" scales below. Your partner should do the same with his or her ratings of you. Again, your partner should use a circle for himself or herself and a square for you.

When finished, you will have a graphic representation of the changes.

NURTURING

1   2   3   4   5   6   7   8   9   10

SENSUALITY

1   2   3   4   5   6   7   8   9   10

SELF-IMAGE

1   2   3   4   5   6   7   8   9   10

SELF-DEFINITION

1   2   3   4   5   6   7   8   9   10

COMFORT

1   2   3   4   5   6   7   8   9   10

KNOWLEDGE

1   2   3   4   5   6   7   8   9   10

RELATIONSHIP

1   2   3   4   5   6   7   8   9   10

PARTNERS

1   2   3   4   5   6   7   8   9   10

NONGENITAL SEX

1   2   3   4   5   6   7   8   9   10

GENITAL SEX

1   2   3   4   5   6   7   8   9   10

SPIRITUALITY

1   2   3   4   5   6   7   8   9   10

PASSION

1   2   3   4   5   6   7   8   9   10

After completing the combined scales, answer the following questions, and then share your answers with your partner and fair witnesses. (See the debriefing exercise on page 358.)

1. In what areas have you progressed and grown?

2. In what areas do you still need more work?

3. In what areas have your perceptions of yourself and your partner's perceptions of you become more similar?

   In what areas do these perceptions remain dissimilar?

4. In what areas have your perceptions of your partner and your partner's perceptions of himself or herself become more similar?

   In what areas do these perceptions remain dissimilar?

APPENDIX A

The Twelve Dimensions, Strategies, and Principles of Healthy Sexuality

Dimensions of Healthy Sexuality

1. NURTURING—the capacity to receive care from others and provide care for self.

2. SENSUALITY—the mindfulness of physical senses that creates emotional, intellectual, spiritual, and physical presence.

3. SELF-IMAGE—a positive self-perception that includes embracing your sexual self.

4. SELF-DEFINITION—a clear knowledge of yourself, both positive and negative, and the ability to express boundaries as well as needs.

Supportive Strategies

1. SEEK MODELS OF NURTURING and note how they apply to our sexuality. Plan specific ways to nurture self and allow others to nurture us. In general, to practice acceptance and self-care.

2. DETERMINE WHAT RULES prevent you from being sensual and focused on the present. Plan concrete and specific ways to notice what your senses are telling you. Integrate your sense awareness into your sexual imagery.

3. ASK WHAT WERE THE AGENDAS of the original "programmers" of your sexuality; discover which no longer fit in your life, and what help you can get now. Construct new sexual affirmations.

4. BEGIN TAKING A STAND about who you are as a sexual person. Clarify sexual priorities and set boundaries so that you can be safe and sexual. Cultivate discernment through daily meditation, reading, and sensual attunement.

12 Step Principles

1. THE FIRST STEP asks us to let others care for us and to learn to take care of ourselves. This means giving up control, letting go, and trusting others.

2. THE SECOND STEP reminds us that an awareness of little things helps us to trust that there are larger forces at work in our lives. A sense of wonder emerges if we are present to our lives.

3. THE THIRD STEP underlines the leap of faith necessary to believe in ourselves. The time-honored "act as if" principle assumes a Higher Power who made us lovable and sexual.

4. THE FOURTH STEP asks a "fearless" inventory of who we are which demands a more honest expression of our needs.

Dimensions of Healthy Sexuality	Supportive Strategies	12 Step Principles
5. COMFORT—the capacity to be at ease about sexual matters with oneself and with others.	5. CREATE GREATER COMFORT ABOUT SEX by identifying and overcoming negative and dysfunctional family, religious, and cultural messages about sex. Confronting issues of sexual preferences. Resolving issues created by sexual abuse.	5. THE FIFTH STEP helps us to be fully known by others, including all of our "dark side." This helps us to be comfortable to integrate those pieces we used to hide.
6. KNOWLEDGE—a knowledge base about sex in general and about one's own unique sexual patterns.	6. PAY ATTENTION to the many ways sexual issues enter and affect your day-to-day life. Learn more about sexuality. Operate on the basis of information, not "rules." Develop a plan to learn more about your sexual self.	6. THE SIXTH STEP encourages us to look deeper for "holes" or areas that need work in our life. Some of our most important lessons come to us here.
7. RELATIONSHIP—a capacity to have intimacy and friendship with both those of the same gender and opposite gender.	7. EXAMINE YOUR OWN BELIEFS about men and women. Develop deeper relationships with those of both genders. Learn to separate the erotic from relationships with those of the gender to which you are attracted. Identify those in your life who support your efforts to change.	7. THE SEVENTH STEP allows us to take another leap of faith that these more difficult issues will also be overcome. Working them out adds to our spiritual and life experience.

Dimensions of Healthy Sexuality	Supportive Strategies	12 Step Principles
8. PARTNERSHIP—the ability to maintain an interdependent, equal relationship that is intimate and erotic.	8. EXPLORE HOW THE PRINCIPLES OF HEALTHY SEXUALITY can change the rules of abandonment. Seek out tools to confront sexual exploitation and sexualized conflicts, needs, and self-destructive patterns. Learn and practice behaviors which build and enhance enduring relationships.	8. THE EIGHTH STEP demands a "rigorous" honesty which becomes central to healthy relationships. This honesty makes all relationships durable and our sexual relationship renewable in its eroticism.
9. NONGENITAL SEX—the ability to express erotic desire emotionally and physically without the use of the genitals.	9. LEARN MORE ABOUT NONGENITAL TOUCH, and plan time to enjoy its pleasures. Practice communicating needs and desires; express what feels good. Reduce focus on orgasm; increase focus on the whole process of sex. Use touch to gradually acclimatize self to more fearful levels of sexual contact.	9. THE NINTH STEP is the action step that requires us to do what we can to keep our relationships in order. That means to use all means that we can and to make amends for those areas in which we have not done enough. It also means that when we stop over important parts like nongenital expression, we can make up for it.
10. GENITAL SEX—the ability to freely express erotic feelings with the use of the genitals.	10. IDENTIFY AND WORK THROUGH PROBLEMS of control and power in sex. Confront impotence and pre-orgasmic conditions. Review resources on sexual information and techniques. Choose some new sexual techniques, and make a plan for experimenting with them.	10. THE TENTH STEP builds on the principles of the previous nine and asks that these principles be practiced in our lives. Few activities demand the integration of these principles more than the use of the genitals.

Dimensions of Healthy Sexuality	Supportive Strategies	12 Step Principles
11. SPIRITUALITY—the ability to connect sexual desire and expression to the value and meaning of one's life.	11. SEEK OUT MODELS for creating and communicating meaning in sex. Acknowledge the link between sexuality and spirituality. Examine sexual history to determine where you find meaning in sex. Learn to communicate meaning concurrently and consistently.	11. THE ELEVENTH STEP encourages us to constantly improve our spiritual consciousness. In that way, we remember our connectedness and purpose.
12. PASSION—the capacity to express deeply held feelings of desire and meaning about one's sexual self, relationships, and intimacy experience.	12. STATE PUBLICLY HOW YOU HAVE CHANGED as a result of this process. Publicly witness your "conversion"—your new beliefs, values, and ways of living. Leave the "observer of life" status and actively participate in the world around you.	12. THE TWELFTH STEP asks that we bear witness to our experience to others. Given the centrality of sex in our lives, this includes sexual experiences as well.

APPENDIX B

Appendix B

The Twelve Steps of Alcoholics Anonymous*

1. We admitted we were powerless over alcohol—that our lives had become unmanageable.
2. Came to believe that a Power greater than ourselves could restore us to sanity.
3. Made a decision to turn our will and our lives over to the care of God *as we understood Him.*
4. Made a searching and fearless moral inventory of ourselves.
5. Admitted to God, to ourselves, and to another human being the exact nature of our wrongs.
6. Were entirely ready to have God remove all these defects of character.
7. Humbly asked Him to remove our shortcomings.
8. Made a list of all persons we had harmed, and became willing to make amends to them all.
9. Made direct amends to such people wherever possible, except when to do so would injure them or others.
10. Continued to take personal inventory and when we were wrong promptly admitted it.
11. Sought through prayer and meditation to improve our conscious contact with God *as we understood Him*, praying only for knowledge of His will for us and the power to carry that out.
12. Having had a spiritual awakening as the result of these steps, we tried to carry this message to alcoholics, and to practice these principles in all our affairs.

*The Twelve Steps of AA are taken from Alcoholics Anonymous, 3d ed., published by AA World Services, Inc., New York, N.Y., 59-60. Reprinted with permission of AA World Services, Inc. (See editor's note on copyright page.)

Appendix B

The Twelve Steps of Sex Addicts Anonymous *

1. We admitted we were powerless over our compulsive sexual behavior—that our lives had become unmanageable.
2. Came to believe that a Power greater than ourselves could restore us to sanity.
3. Made a decision to turn our will and lives over to the care of God as we understood God.
4. Made a searching and fearless moral inventory of ourselves.
5. Admitted to God, to ourselves, and to another human being the exact nature of our wrongs.
6. Were entirely ready to have God remove all these defects of character.
7. Humbly asked God to remove our shortcomings.
8. Made a list of all persons we had harmed and became willing to make amends to them all.
9. Made direct amends to such people wherever possible, except when to do so would injure them or others.
10. Continued to take personal inventory and when we were wrong promptly admitted it.
11. Sought through prayer and meditation to improve our conscious contact with God, as we understood God, praying only for knowledge of God's will for us and the power to carry that out.
12. Having had a spiritual awakening as a result of these Steps, we tried to carry this message to sex addicts and to practice these principles in all of our activities.

*Adapted from the Twelve Steps of Alcoholics Anonymous and reprinted with permission of AA World Services, Inc., New York, NY.

Appendix B

The Twelve Steps of Sexaholics Anonymous*

1. We admitted that we were powerless over lust—that our lives had become unmanageable.
2. Came to believe that a Power greater than ourselves could restore us to sanity.
3. Made a decision to turn our will and our lives over to the care of God *as we understood Him.*
4. Made a searching and fearless moral inventory of ourselves.
5. Admitted to God, to ourselves, and to another human being the exact nature of our wrongs.
6. Were entirely ready to have God remove all these defects of character.
7. Humbly asked Him to remove our shortcomings.
8. Made a list of all persons we had harmed, and became willing to make amends to them all.
9. Made direct amends to such people wherever possible, except when to do so would injure them or others.
10. Continued to take personal inventory and when we were wrong promptly admitted it.
11. Sought through prayer and meditation to improve our conscious contact with God *as we understood Him,* praying only for knowledge of His will for us and the power to carry that out.
12. Having had a spiritual awakening as the result of these Steps, we tried to carry this message to sexaholics and to practice these principles in all our affairs.

*Adapted from the Twelve Steps of Alcoholics Anonymous and reprinted with permission of AA World Services, Inc. New York, NY. Copyright © 1989 SA Literature. Reprinted with permission of SA Literature. Permission to reprint does not imply SA affiliation or SA's review or endorsement of this publication.

Appendix B

The Twelve Steps of Sex and Love Addicts Anonymous*

1. We admitted we were powerless over sex and love addiction—that our lives had become unmanageable.
2. Came to believe that a Power greater than ourselves could restore us to sanity.
3. Made a decision to turn our will and lives over to the care of God as we understood God.
4. Made a searching and fearless moral inventory of ourselves.
5. Admitted to God, to ourselves, and to another human being the exact nature of our wrongs.
6. Were entirely ready to have God remove all these defects of character.
7. Humbly asked God to remove our shortcomings.
8. Made a list of all persons we had harmed, and became willing to make amends to them all.
9. Made direct amends to such people wherever possible, except when to do so would injure them or others.
10. Continued to take personal inventory, and when we were wrong promptly admitted it.
11. Sought through prayer and meditation to improve our conscious contact with a Power greater than ourselves, praying only for knowledge of God's will for us and the power to carry that out.
12. Having had a spiritual awakening as a result of these steps, we tried to carry this message to sex and love addicts, and to practice these principles in all areas of our lives.

*Adapted from the Twelve Steps of Alcoholics Anonymous and reprinted with permission of AA World Services, Inc., New York, NY. Reprinted with the permission of The Augustine Fellowship, Sex and Love Addicts Anonymous.

The Twelve Suggested Steps of Sexual Compulsives Anonymous*

1. We admitted we were powerless over sexual compulsion—that our lives had become unmanageable.
2. Came to believe that a power greater than ourselves could restore us to sanity.
3. Made a decision to turn our will and our lives over to the care of God, *as we understood God.*
4. Made a searching and fearless moral inventory of ourselves.
5. Admitted to God, to ourselves, and to another human being the exact nature of our wrongs.
6. Were entirely ready to have God remove all these defects of character.
7. Humbly asked God to remove our shortcomings.
8. Made a list of all persons we had harmed and became willing to make amends to them all.
9. Made direct amends to such people wherever possible, except when to do so would injure them or others.
10. Continued to take personal inventory and when we were wrong promptly admitted it.
11. Sought through prayer and meditation to improve our conscious contact with God, *as we understood God*, praying only for knowledge of God's will for us and the power to carry that out.
12. Having had a spiritual awakening as the result of these steps, we tried to carry this message to sexually compulsive people, and to practice these principles in all our affairs.

---

*Adapted from the Twelve Steps of Alcoholics Anonymous and reprinted with permission of AA World Services, Inc., New York, NY. The Twelve Suggested Steps of SCA are taken from *Sexual Compulsives Anonymous: A Program of Recovery*, published by International Service Organization of Sexual Compulsives Anonymous, New York, N.Y., p. 2. Reprinted with permission.

INTRODUCTION

1. For professionals the literature comparing extremes in food and sex can be found most recently in Helen Kaplan Singer's *The Sexual Desire Disorders* (New York: Brunner/Mazel, 1995), 19. For an early summary of the literature and a thoughtful comparison of food and sexual anorexia see R. Hardman, and D. Gardner "Sexual Anorexia: A Look at Inhibited Sexual Desire," *Journal of Sex Education and Therapy* 12 (1): 55–59.

CHAPTER 1: SEX AS FUNDMENTAL

1. Rudolph M. Bell, *Holy Anorexia* (Chicago: University of Chicago Press, 1985).
2. For information, see Patrick Carnes, *Don't Call It Love* (New York: Bantam, 1993).
3. For information on the addictive patterns in food use, see L. L'Abate, J. Farran, and D. Serritelia, eds., *Handbook of Differential Treatments of Addiction* (Boston: Allyn and Bacon, 1992).
4. Hans Heubner, Endorphins, *Eating Disorders and Other Addictive Behaviors* (New York: W. W. Norton, 1993).
5. *Diagnostic and Statistical Manual of Mental Disorders*, 4th ed. (Washington, D.C.: American Psychiatric Association, 1994).
6. For a review of the language problems across the involved disciplines see Patrick Carnes, "Sexual Addiction or Compulsion: Politics or Illness?" *Sexual Addiction and Compulsivity, The Journal of Treatment and Prevention* (1996).
7. "The Ebb and Flow of Sexual Desire," *Sex Over Forty*, Nov. 1993, quoting *U.S. News & World Report*.
8. L. DeMause, "The Universality of Incest," *Journal of Psychohistory* 19 (1991): 123–64.
9. For sources on this data, see Stephanie Coontz, *The Way We Never Were* (New York: Basic Books, 1992); John N. Briere, *Child Abuse Trauma: Theory and Treatment of the Lasting Effects* (Newbury Park, Calif.: Sage Publications, 1992); *Carnes Update* (Summer 1995).
10. R. Sipe, *Sex, Priests and Power* (New York: Brunner/Mazel, 1995).
11. Gordon L. Benson, "Sexual Behavior by Male Clergy with Adult Female Counselees: Systemic and Situational Themes," *Sexual Addiction and Compulsivity* 1, no. 2 (1994): 103–18.
12. "U.S. Leads in Child Homicides," *Arizona Republic*, 7 February 1997.

13. Peter Gay, *The Bourgeois Experience—Victoria to Freud*, vol. 1 of *Education of the Senses* (New York: Oxford University Press, 1984).

14. L. DeMause, "The History of Child Abuse," *Sexual Addiction and Compulsivity* 1, no. 1 (1994).

15. L. DeMause, "The History of Child Abuse."

16. L. DeMause, "The History of Child Abuse."

17. Denise Breton and Christopher Largent, *The Paradigm Conspiracy: How Our Systems of Government, Church, School & Culture Violate Our Human Potential* (Center City, Minn.: Hazelden, 1996), 285.

CHAPTER 2: SEX AS DEPRIVATION

1. Hung-chih Cheng-chueh quoted and translated by Robert Aiken in "The Middle Way," in *Parabola,* 12, no. 2, p. 40. This was a special issue on addiction issues.

2. Aline Rouselle, Porneia: *On Desire and the Body in Antiquity* (New York: Basil Blackwell, 1988).

CHAPTER 3: SEX AS EXTREME

1. Sex and Love Addicts Anonymous, *Anorexia: Sexual, Social, Emotional* (W. Newton, Mass.: The Augustine Fellowship, 1992).

2. Merle A. Fossum and Marilyn J. Mason, *Facing Shame: Families in Recovery* (New York: Norton, 1986), 105–22.

3. Erik Erikson, *Identity and the Life Cycle* (New York: Norton, 1980).

4. Alayne Yates, *Compulsive Exercise and the Eating Disorders* (New York: Brunner/Mazel, 1991).

5. Domeena Renshaw, *Medical Aspects of Human Sexuality* (April 1990). See also Sharon Klayman Farber, "Research paper" (Ph.D. diss., New York University, May 1995).

6. A. J. Yellowlees, "Anorexia and Bulimia in Anorexia Nervosa: A Study of Psychosocial Functioning and Associated Psychiatric Symptomology," *British Journal of Psychiatry* (1985): 146, 648–52.

7. Sandra L. Bloom, "Every Time History Repeats Itself, the Price Goes Up: The Social Reenactment of Trauma," *Sexual Addiction and Compulsivity* 3, no. 3 (1986).

8. June Butts, "The Relationship between Sexual Addiction and Sexual Dysfunction," *Journal of Health Care for the Poor and Underserved* 3, no. 1 (1992); Barry W. McCarthy, "Sexually Compulsive Men and Inhibited Sexual Desire," *Journal of Sex and Marital Therapy* 20, no. 3 (1994).

9. Charles Moser, "Lust, Lack of Desire, and Paraphilias: Some Thoughts and Possible Connections," *Journal of Sex and Marital Therapy* 18, no. 1 (1992); P. deSilva, "Fetishism and Sexual Dysfunction: Clinical Presentation and Management," *Journal of Sex and Marital Therapy* 8, no. 3 (1993): 147–55.

10. Ian T. Bownes and Ethna C. O'Gorman, "Assailants' Sexual Dysfunction during Rape Reported by Their Victims," *Medicine, Science, and the Law* 31, no. 4 (October 1991): 322–28; Eugene J. Kanin, "Date Rapists: Differential Sexual Socialization and Relative Deprivation," *Archives of Sexual Behavior* 14, no. 3 (June 1985): 219–31.

11. Jennifer Schneider, *Back from Betrayal: Recover from His Affairs* (San Francisco: Harper and Row, 1988).

CHAPTER 5: SEX AS HEALTH

1. Paul Watzlawick, John Weakland, and Richard Risch, *Change: Principles of Problem Formation and Problem Resolution* (New York: W. W. Norton and Co., 1974).

2. Stephen Covey, *The Seven Habits of Highly Effective People* (New York: Simon and Schuster, 1989).

3. James Maddock, "Healthy Family Sexuality: Positive Principles for Educators and Clinicians," *Family Relations* 38 (April 1989): 130–36.

4. Ginger Manley, "Sexual Health Recovery in Sex Addictions: Implications for Sex Therapists," *American Journal of Preventive Psychiatry and Neurology* 3, no. 2 (1991).

5. Sharon Day, "American Indian Sexuality: Our Own Definitions," VIEWS, Minnesota Association for the Education of Young Children (Summer 1993).

CHAPTER 7: SENSUALITY

1. Philippe Aries, *The Hour of Our Death*, trans. Helen Weaver (New York: Knopf, 1981).

2. Based on exercises in Bernard Gunther, *Sense Relaxation* (North Hollywood, Calif.: Newcastle, 1986).

CHAPTER 9: SELF-DEFINITION

1. Erik Erikson, *Identity and the Life Cycle* (New York: W. W. Norton, 1980).

2. Henri Nouwen, *Reaching Out: The Three Movements of the Spiritual Life* (New York: Doubleday, 1986).

3. M. Scott Peck, *The Road Less Traveled* (New York: Simon and Schuster,

CHAPTER 10: SEXUAL COMFORT

1. Wendy Maltz, *The Sexual Healing Journey: A Guide for Survivors of Sexual Abuse* (New York: HarperCollins, 1995), 6-7.

CHAPTER 11: KNOWLEDGE

1. William Masters and Virginia Johnson, *Masters and Johnson on Sex and Human Loving* (New York: Little, Brown, 1986), 263-81.
2. See, for example,William Betcher, *Intimate Play: Creating Romance in Everyday Life* (New York: Viking Penguin, 1988), 140-46
3. Joseph Nowinski, *Men Love & Sex: A Couple's Guide to Male Sexual Fulfillment* (San Francisco: Thorsons, 1991).
4. "The Ten Most Common Questions Men Ask about Sex" and "The Ten Most Common Questions Women Ask about Sex," adapted from the *Sex Over Forty* newsletter of December 1991, January 1993, June 1993, and July 1993. Used with permission.

CHAPTER 13: PARTNERS

1. M. Scott Peck, *Further Along the Road Less Traveled* (New York: Simon and Schuster, 1993).
2. Patrick J. Carnes, *Don't Call It Love* (New York: Bantam Books, 1991).
3. A. H. Maslow, *Motivation and Personality* (New York: Harper & Row, 1970).
4. Erich Fromm, *Man for Himself* (New York: Holt, 1990), 129-30.
5. A. H. Maslow, *Motivation and Personality*.
6. J. Richard Conkerly and Kathleen A. McClaren, "Love Behavior Training for Sex Counselors and Therapists: A Way Toward Improvement?" *Journal of Sex Education and Therapy* 12 (Spring/Summer 1986).
7. J. Richard Conkerly and Kathleen A. McClaren, "Sex Therapy with and without Love: An Empirical Investigation," *Journal of Sex Education and Therapy* 8 (Fall/Winter 1982).

CHAPTER 14: NONGENITAL SEX

1. *Sex over 40* (January 1993).
2. Wendy Maltz,*The Sexual Healing Journey: A Guide for Survivors of Sexual Abuse* (New York: HarperCollins, 1995), 251-85.

CHAPTER 15: GENITAL SEX

1. Wendy Maltz, *The Sexual Healing Journey: A Guide for Survivors of Sexual Abuse* (New York: HarperCollins, 1995).
2. Ibid.

CHAPTER 17: PASSION

1. Marilyn Murray, *Prisoner of Another War* (Berkeley, Calif.: Page Mill Press, 1991).

RECOMMENDED RESOURCES

Books

Anand, Margo. *The Art of Sexual Ecstasy: The Path of Sacred Sexuality for Western Lovers.* Los Angeles: J. P. Tarcher, 1989.

Aries, Philippe. *The Hour of Our Death.* Trans. Helen Weaver. New York: Knopf, 1981.

Becker, Ernest. *The Denial of Death.* New York: Free Press, 1985.

Betcher, William. *Intimate Play: Creating Romance in Everyday Life.* New York: Viking Penguin, 1988.

Bradshaw, John. *Creating Love: The Next Great Stage of Growth.* New York: Bantam Books, 1994.

Breton, Denise, and Christopher Largent. *The Paradigm Conspiracy: How Our Systems of Government, Church, School, and Culture Violate Our Human Potential.* Center City, Minn.: Hazelden, 1996.

Cameron, Julia. *The Artist's Way.* New York: Putnam, 1995.

Campbell, Joseph. *The Hero with a Thousand Faces.* Princeton, N.J.: Princeton University Press, 1990.

Covington, Stephanie. *Awakening Your Sexuality: A Guide for Recovering Women.* San Francisco: Harper, 1992.

Davis, Laura. *Allies in Healing: When the Person You Love Was Sexually Abused as a Child.* New York: HarperCollins, 1991.

Erikson, Erik. *Identity, Youth, and Crisis.* New York: W. W. Norton, 1968.

Fromm, Erich. *Man for Himself.* New York: Holt, 1990.

Godek, Gregory J. P. *1001 Ways to Be Romantic.* Weymouth, Mass.: Casablanca Press, 1995.

Gunther, Bernard. *Sense Relaxation.* North Hollywood, Calif.: Newcastle, 1986.

Hastings, Anne S. *Discovering Sexuality That Will Satisfy You Both: When Couples Want Differing Amounts and Different Kinds of Sex.* Tiburon, Calif.: Printed Voice, 1993.

Henderson, Julie. *The Lover Within: Opening to Energy in Sexual Practice.* Barrytown, N.Y.: Station Hill Press, 1987.

Hunter, Mic. *Joyous Sexuality: Healing from the Effects of Family Sexual Dysfunction.* Minneapolis: CompCare, 1992.

Resources

Klausner, Mary Ann, and Bobbie Hasselbring. *Aching for Love: The Sexual Drama of the Adult Child: Healing Strategies for Women.* San Francisco: Harper & Row, 1990.

Kraft, William F. *Whole and Holy Sexuality.* Saint Meinrad, Ind.: Abbey Press, 1989.

Lewis, Helen Block. *Psychic War in Men and Women.* New York: New York University Press, 1976.

Liebowitz, Michael R. *The Chemistry of Love.* Boston: Little, Brown, 1982.

Louden, Jennifer. *The Couple's Comfort Book: A Creative Guide for Renewing Passion, Pleasure and Commitment.* San Francisco: Harper, 1994.

Love, Patricia. *Emotional Incest Syndrome: What to Do When a Parent's Love Rules Your Life.* New York: Bantam Books, 1991.

Love, Patricia, and Jo Robinson. *Hot Monogamy: Essential Steps to More Passionate, Intimate Lovemaking.* New York: Dutton, 1995.

Maltz, Wendy. *The Sexual Healing Journey: A Guide for Survivors of Sexual Abuse.* New York: HarperCollins, 1995.

——————. *Passionate Hearts.* San Rafael, Calif.: New World Library, 1997.

Maslow, A. H. *Motivation and Personality.* New York: HarperCollins, 1987.

Masters, William H., and Virginia E. Johnson. *Masters and Johnson on Sex and Human Loving.* New York: Little, Brown, 1988.

Mellody, Pia, et al. *Facing Love Addiction: Giving Yourself the Power to Change the Way You Love.* San Francisco: Harper, 1992.

Morin, Jack. *Erotic Mind: Unlocking the Inner Sources of Sexual Passion and Fulfillment.* New York: HarperCollins, 1996.

Nelson, James B. *Embodiment: An Approach to Sexuality and Christian Theology.* Minneapolis: Augsburg Fortress, 1979.

Nouwen, Henri. *Reaching Out: The Three Movements of the Spiritual Life.* New York: Doubleday, 1986.

Nowinski, Joseph. *Men, Love, and Sex.* San Francisco: Thorsons, 1991.

Peck, M. Scott. *The Road Less Traveled: A New Psychology of Love, Traditional Values and Spiritual Growth.* New York: Simon and Schuster, 1980.

Schnarch, David M. *Constructing the Sexual Crucible.* New York: W. W. Norton, 1991.

Resources

Sears, Berry. *The Zone*. New York: HarperCollins, 1995.

Simon, Sidney B. *Values Clarification: A Handbook of Practical Strategies for Teachers and Students*. Sunderland, Mass.: Values Press, 1991.

Newsletters

Sex over 40: A Practical, Authoritative Newsletter Directed to the Sexual Concerns of the Mature Adult. DKT International, P. O. Box 1600, Chapel Hill, NC 27515.

Erotic Instructional Videos

The Better Sex Video Series has already sold close to one million copies in the United States. Volumes include *Better Sexual Techniques; Advanced Sexual Techniques, Making Sex Fun; Guide to Oral Sex;* and *You Can Last Longer.*

The Sinclair Institute offers three videotapes: *Speaking of Sex; Sexual Positions for Lovers;* and *Becoming Orgasmic.*

Loving Better is a five-volume series featuring *The Basics; Discovery* (focusing on sense exercises); *Loving and Caring; Enhancement; and Sexual Problems.*

All can be ordered from *Sex over 40* by calling 1-800-285-0444.

For information on Education, Newsletters, and Conferences call the National Council on Sexual Addiction and Compulsion:

National Council on Sexual Addiction & Compulsivity (NCSAC)
1090 Northchase Parkway, Suite 200 South
Marietta, GA 30067
(770) 989-9754

For specific 12 Step Groups on Sex Addiction:

Sex and Love Addicts Anonymous (SLAA)
P.O. Box 650010, 437 Cherry Street
West Newton, MA 02165-0010
(617) 332-1845

(Most common on East and West Coast)

Sexaholics Anonymous (SA)
P.O. Box 111910
Nashville, TN 37222-1910
(615) 331-6230

(Throughout the country but not as common)

Sex Addicts Anonymous (SAA)
P.O. Box 3038
Minneapolis, MN 55403
(612) 339-0217 or (713) 869-4902

(Most common and especially strong through the middle of the country)

Sexual Compulsive Anonymous (SCA)
P.O. Box, 1585 Old Chelsea Station
New York, NY 10011
(212) 439-1123 or (213) 896-2964, in Los Angeles, CA (310) 859-5585

(For gay and lesbian people all over the county)

Recovering Couples Anonymous (RCA)
P.O. Box 11872
St. Louis, MO 63105
(314) 830-2600

National Council for Couple and Family Recovery (NCCFR)
(Jim & Mary Lane)
434 Lee Avenue
St. Louis, MO 63119
(314) 963-8898

For certified therapists in your city, call The Meadows at 1-800-MEADOWS or 1-800-632-3697

Index

Index

Index

Index

Index

Index

About the Author

Patrick J. Carnes, Ph.D., C.A.S., is a nationally known authority on addiction and recovery issues. He is the author of *Out of the Shadows: Understanding Sexual Addiction; Contrary to Love: Helping the Sexual Addict; A Gentle Path through the Twelve Steps: For All People in the Process of Recovery;* and *Don't Call It Love: Recovery from Sexual Addiction.* His first book on family systems, *Understanding Us*, is regarded as a classic in family education.

Dr. Carnes is the clinical director for sexual disorder services at the Meadows in Wickenburg, Arizona. Additionally, he is the editor-in-chief of *Sexual Addiction and Compulsivity: The Journal of Treatment and Prevention*, the official journal of the National Council of Sexual Addiction/Compulsivity.

Dr. Carnes received a Bachelor of Arts degree from St. John's University, Collegeville, Minnesota, a Master's degree from Brown University, and a Doctorate in Counselor Education and Organizational Development from the University of Minnesota.

HAZELDEN INFORMATION AND EDUCATIONAL SERVICES is a division of the Hazelden Foundation, a not-for-profit organization. Since 1949, Hazelden has been a leader in promoting the dignity and treatment of people afflicted with the disease of chemical dependency.

The mission of the foundation is to improve the quality of life for individuals, families, and communities by providing a national continuum of information, education, and recovery services that are widely accessible; to advance the field through research and training; and to improve our quality and effectiveness through continuous improvement and innovation.

Stemming from that, the mission of this division is to provide quality information and support to people wherever they may be in their personal journey—from education and early intervention, through treatment and recovery, to personal and spiritual growth.

Although our treatment programs do not necessarily use everything Hazelden publishes, our bibliotherapeutic materials support our mission and the Twelve Step philosophy upon which it is based. We encourage your comments and feedback.

The headquarters of the Hazelden Foundation are in Center City, Minnesota. Additional treatment facilities are located in Chicago, Illinois; New York, New York; Plymouth, Minnesota; St. Paul, Minnesota; and West Palm Beach, Florida. At these sites, we provide a continuum of care for men and women of all ages. Our Plymouth facility is designed specifically for youth and families.

For more information on Hazelden, please call **1-800-257-7800.** Or you may access our World Wide Web site on the Internet at **http://www.hazelden.org.**